P9-BZA-166

"A new book to be read is by Dr. Scott Fried. It sets up patient guidelines on how to understand and deal with Neuropathies of the median, ulnar, radial and Brachial Plexus nerves of the hand and upper extremity. *Light at the End of the Carpal Tunnel* is fun, readable and very informative. It fills a need in the nerve gap in a doctor/patient relationship."

James M. Hunter, M.D.
Distinguished Professor of Orthopaedic (Hand) Surgery
Jefferson Medical College of the
Thomas Jefferson University
Philadelphia, PA

LIGHT
at the End of the
Carpal Tunnel

*A Guide to Understanding
and Relief from the
Pain of Nerve Problems*

Dr. Scott M. Fried

Healing Books
East Norriton, PA 19401

Copyright © 1998 Scott M. Fried. Printed and bound in the United States of America. All rights reserved. No part of this book may be reproduced or transmitted in any form or by any means, electronic or mechanical, including photocopying, recording, or by an information storage and retrieval system—except by a reviewer who may quote brief passages in a review to be printed in a magazine or newspaper—without permission in writing from the publisher. For information, please contact Healing Books, 180 West Germantown Pike, Suite B1A, East Norriton, PA 19401.

MEDICAL DISCLAIMER: Although the authors, editors, and publishers have made every effort to ensure the accuracy and completeness of information contained in this book, it is difficult to ensure that all of the information is accurate and the possibility of error can never be entirely eliminated. The authors, editors, and publishers disclaim any liability or responsibility for injury or damage to persons or property which is incurred as a consequence, directly or indirectly, of the use and application of any of the contents of this book as well as for any unintentional slights to any person or entity. It is the reader's responsibility to know and follow local care protocol as provided by the medical advisors directing the system to which he or she belongs. Also, it is the reader's responsibility to stay informed of changes in the treatment of upper extremity injuries. Medicine is an ever changing science. As new research and clinical experience broaden our knowledge, changes of treatment are required. The author, editors, and the publishers of this work have checked with sources believed to be reliable in their efforts to provide information that is complete and generally in accord with the standards accepted at the time of publication. However, in view of the possibility of human error or changes in medical science, neither the editors, authors, or publishers, nor any other party who has been involved in the preparation of or publication of this work warrant that the information contained herein is in every respect accurate or complete and they are not responsible for any errors, omissions, inaccuracies, inconsistencies, misrepresentations or for the results obtained from the use of such information. Readers are encouraged to confirm the information contained herein with other sources.

First printing 1998

ISBN 0-9659267-5-3

LCCN 97-094105

Editing, design, typesetting, and printing services provided by About Books, Inc., 425 Cedar Street, POB 1500, Buena Vista, CO 81211, (800) 548-1876.

ATTENTION CORPORATIONS, UNIVERSITIES, COLLEGES, AND PROFESSIONAL ORGANIZATIONS: Quantity discounts are available on bulk purchases of this book for educational purposes. Special books or book excerpts can also be created to fit specific needs. For information, please contact Healing Books, 180 West Germantown Pike, Suite B1A, East Norriton, PA 19401. Phone 610-277-1998 or fax 610-277-2007.

CONTENTS

ACKNOWLEDGMENTS

When I actually put my pen to paper to write my book on carpal tunnel and complex nerve problems, my greatest insight came from the most unexpected sources. My children, Joshua and Allison, have reached the age where their playful yet intense curiosity and thirst for knowledge have become the overwhelming issue in our lives. It seems children have a wonderful ability to get to the heart of matters and directly to the point. If I hurt my daughter's feelings, she simply looks at me with her big green eyes and says, "Daddy, you hurt my feelings." Joshua, on the other hand, has been known to lecture my wife and me in a polite yet concise manner indicating our logic as adults is often clouded by too many other issues.

I remember a specific instance when my then three-year-old nephew accidentally hit Josh in the head with a toy, causing a laceration. My daughter, Allison, immediately recognized the situation and brought to our attention the fact that my son's cries were not just an attention-getting device. When my brother and I saw the blood gushing from his forehead, our worst fears all came to mind. Once the situation was assessed, Joshua calmed us both by assuring us he was not really in pain and it looked worse than it really was.

Before I sutured his head on the living room couch (a doctor's insanity), Joshua took time to gently remind my brother his three-year-old son had no intention of hurting him; this was simply an accident. He stated my brother's admonishments of Jonathan were somewhat overreactive, and when things were put into perspective, this wasn't such a bad deal. Thank God for children, and especially mine, who have given me such wonderful insight into myself and my work.

I certainly would be remiss in not acknowledging those who have given me the insight to understand nerve problems. Although many have taught me, Dr. James Hunter is no doubt the greatest thinker. He is a man whose understanding of nerves and nerve problems goes beyond the accepted and truly into another realm. He has taught me many things about people and medicine, especially that they are related. Dr. Hunter showed me nerves are truly predictable, and if we listen to our patients, they will tell us what is wrong and how to fix it. He has taught me to re-read the works of people such as Sunderland and Roos and has enabled me to realize not only that nerve problems are curable but also that they must be addressed from their true underlying etiology.

Dr. Stephen Whitenack must be recognized for his great technical skills and for imparting these to me as best anyone could. His skill and success with thoracic outlet patients made me a true believer that this problem could be helped surgically. The hours I spent operating with Drs. Hunter and Whitenack were among the most fulfilling and informative in my career.

Drs. Lee Osterman and Scott Jaeger cannot go unmentioned. Dr. Osterman first introduced me to hand surgery many years ago and lit within me a light which continues to burn till this day. Dr. Jaeger gave me great early insight into thoracic outlet and nerve problems and was truly the first to bring me out of the realm of general orthopedic surgeon and into that of hand surgeon. Both, in very different ways, molded much of my early career thinking and direction.

Dr. Bernie Siegel is a true pioneer and great thinker as well. He has reminded us of the true importance of the human being and that the doctor-patient relationship should be valued by patients and their doctors. When I originally read Dr. Siegel's works, I realized he was not simply talking about patients dying from cancer but actually referring to all patients who suffered in any way. In essence he offers help and hope to all who suffer.

I was privileged to have the opportunity to meet Dr. Siegel and also have him review and critique my manuscript. Dr. Siegel's thinking and influences are, as you will see, threaded throughout the chapters of this book. Many of my concepts on healing itself have come from Dr. Siegel and his works, and I thank him for his wonderful insight. I applaud his true bravery as a pioneer who went against the mainstream. He opened the door to those of us who wish to be "doctors" and who love our patients.

Professor Lester Levin is not only my father-in-law but also a true friend. As a teacher and author, he has given me wonderful guidance in putting my book together. His literary recommendations as well as his personal views on many of the issues presented have been not only helpful but key in formulating the basics of the book.

My brother, Rick, a psychologist and dermatologist, has been of great help in moving forward with the aspects of the book that refer to biofeedback and psychology. Rick and I have spent years ruminating over many of the ideas set forth here and as a best friend and brother, his support has always been there to help me move forward.

Chris Leichliter and Frank Murphy have been true lights at the end of my own tunnel. They have helped take my manuscript from coarse to fine through their input, advice, and insight.

I cannot thank them enough for taking on the project and helping to put the book into its fully finished form.

To my good friend and fellow hand surgeon, Miguel Pirela-Cruz, thanks are not enough. His wonderful combination of hand surgical expertise and artistic talent have created pictures to go with my words as only Miguel could do.

What can I say about Maryann? Through the years and the craziness, my secretary, office manager, confidante, and friend has always been there. Whether it's late at night, early in morning, or over the weekend when she should have been at home, Maryann is always there to finish something, re-edit, comment, or rewrite my English. Sometimes I have the feeling this book is as much Maryann's as mine, and I can't thank her enough for her help, support, and friendship.

My mother, Lee Fried, began my philosophy training at a very early age. She is a constant support and source of great intuitive insight into people and possibilities. When things seem impossible, she has the proper words, encouragement, and knowledge to bring things back into perspective and help me move forward through almost any trial, tribulation, or challenge.

My father, Dr. Sidney Fried, is a clinical psychologist and probably the most insightful and benevolent human being whose acquaintance one could ever hope to make. If anyone could ever hope for a role model, he's it. What has amazed me over the years about my father is his unique capacity to love people and even more so his ability to have people love him. He has an innate ability to assess situations, pain, and human behavior. He seems to find mystical paths, changing nightmares into pleasant dreams. This goes beyond medical and psychological expertise into the realm of a sixth sense combined with a pure love of people.

Dan Fogleberg wrote a song called "Leader of the Band" in which he describes himself as "just a living legacy to the leader of the band." No one has done more to shape my life and thinking or contributed more to my thought processes, ideals, and love of mankind than my dad.

When it comes to gaining insight to human beings and human behavior, three of my greatest teachers and helpers are Josh, Allison, and Hannah. My children are truly the light of my life and aside from my wife, Laura, bring me my greatest joys and revelations. Initially, watching them grow was the greatest thrill I could ever hope for. Over the years, I've come to realize they have much more to teach me than I can teach them. Their tenacity, lust for life, and unconditional love are the basis for all strength in human behaviors. Watching them go through daily traumas, hernia operations, mental and physical challenges, and just day-to-day living has taught me that very early on we learn the ability to deal with illness. And, if we don't learn it early in life, it is indeed a difficult thing to teach adults.

To my patients, I must say a word of thanks. You have truly been great teachers and friends. Although there are countless thousands of you, many stand out and have become great friends. The hours spent in the exam rooms, operating rooms, and therapy unit sharing stories, tears, and laughter hold some of the best memories of my life. This book is truly a testament to what you have taught me. It is my privilege to share what I've learned from you.

Last but not least, I thank my wife Laura. It is beyond me why someone so lovely, intelligent, and good-natured would put up with such a crazy human being as myself. When I met Laura, I had not a penny in my pocket and only ideals. When I finally reached the point where I could begin my orthopedic career, I told her I wanted to do yet more training to subspecialize in hand and upper-extremity surgery. Although she really wanted to get on with our lives, she somehow knew this was a good decision and supported me all the way. Over the years,

I've continued to drag her in many different directions and looking back, she may have pushed me in many others. She has always been my greatest support, critic, cheerleader, confidante, advisor, and most of all a loving and supportive friend. In spite of the many years I've put into writing this book, there have been very few, if any, complaints about the time spent away from her and the family. In many ways, this is more her book than mine and many of the ideas set forth here come from Laura. Somehow as a nurse, Laura has a much greater clinical insight to many of the problems and issues I discuss in the book than I do. She is much closer in many ways to patient care and has a wonderful way of keeping our lives and careers in perspective. This book and my achievements would certainly not have been possible without my best friend and partner.

Thank you, Laura, for getting us through this. This book is for you—my other and, no doubt, better half.

PREFACE

When I first made the decision to go into medicine some 20 years ago, it was still a noble profession. As a child, I watched my dad, a clinical psychologist, take care of people. I observed the great satisfaction he obtained from making their lives better. I also lived through the long hours and saw the tremendous dedication it took to practice. There were many nights when the phone would ring at 3:00 A.M., and I truly did not appreciate the meaning of this dedication until I, too, was given the privilege of caring for people.

Unfortunately, today's medicine is no longer the profession it was years ago. This is not due to practitioners' lack of dedication but rather to the ever-increasing constraints and limitations placed on them with respect to their every treatment decision. Gone are the days when a doctor could not only tell a patient what was wrong but could dictate his or her medical treatment. Today, statistics rather than intuition and empathy dictate treatment. If you fall outside of the norm, then frankly, you are flat out of luck.

Patients are not thought of as people anymore but rather as "diseases or CPT code diagnoses." This was exactly the kind of thinking we were taught to avoid in medical school and during training. Unfortunately, this is the thinking being forced upon medical practitioners today. Doctors are told to treat people as statistics, numbers, and labels and not as individuals. This presents an extraordinarily dangerous scenario. When the ability to care daily for patients and make decisions is taken out of the hands of the doctor and given to clerks and statisticians, people get hurt. Discussions center around how doctors can be more efficient and productive. The words "understanding," "caring," and "concern" are not heard anymore. Doctors are not even called doctors but rather "providers." This reminds me of a *Star Trek* episode in which "the providers" had evolved to the point where they had forgotten about human compassion and emotion. Have we really gone that far backward?

In his book *Love, Medicine and Miracles*, Dr. Bernie Siegel talks about his initial discomfort when hugged by his patients. Later he learned to hug them back. This became very much a part of the patient's and Siegel's healing process. Dr. Siegel says most of us lack enough love in our lives. But when someone expresses this love, and especially a person of authority, the healing process proceeds at a more rapid and efficient pace.

Why am I writing this book? It is for all those people who have fallen through the cracks of the medical system. This book is for those who have never had the opportunity to visit with a doctor who understood their unique pain and problems. It is for those who never had the opportunity to shed tears of relief when they found out that indeed they were not crazy for all the pain, symptoms, and emotions they had been feeling. It is for all those who have been told they are crazy because the surgery "failed." These patients were never told it was not because of their failure they continued to have symptoms but rather a failure of diagnosis.

The sin and the essence of what I have termed the "carpal tunnel syndrome" is that the syndrome itself is not a disease but rather a disease process of our society today. It stems from lack of respect for people as patients and human beings and the underlying physiologic basis for their pain. More than 500,000 carpal tunnel surgeries were performed in the United States last year. Many of these patients continue to suffer.

What this syndrome is really about is that we have forgotten nerves start at the neck and end at the fingertips. It's about the constraints of medicine today and the fact that doctors as well as patients are influenced by so many factors that the patient's suffering becomes the last issue of concern.

I continue to be amazed and appalled that many patients are never completely diagnosed. I see patients still in pain after being treated for their "carpal tunnel problem," yet no one has ever looked beyond the wrist or hand to see if there is another cause for their pain. Symptoms are classically *not* carpal tunnel and yet they undergo this surgery. People are subjected to operations, injections, medications, and regimens based on suppositions rather than on confirmed diagnoses. I have seen patients who have been in and out of pain programs for years and told there was no physiologic basis for their pain. In fact, these people not only had a diagnosable disease but treatable processes which ultimately resulted in their pain and "psychosis."

So what is the carpal tunnel syndrome? It is simply a mistaken state of mind in our society that treats real pain and real disease of many causes and etiologies as a "simple problem" with an easy cure. In fact, this could not be further from the truth. Carpal tunnel problems are just one segment of a complex group of nerve problems prominent today caused by changes in industry, transportation, and traumas inflicted on ourselves by a highly stressed and highly motivated society. Understanding this problem and the reality of this situation is the first step we must take to overcome the myths and prejudices so prevalent today and which result in severe pain and suffering to many unknowing, innocent individuals. Because of my concern and also my inherent faith in the patients I have met and who have taught me, I decided to write this book. There is no doubt if a person is educated about the problems he or she has, that person can essentially dictate his or her own medical treatment. If a patient understands the basic concept of what is wrong with him or her, then the patient can at least be qualified to determine if judgments are being made in his best interest or strictly based on statistics, numbers, or lack of understanding. I reached the point where I not only wanted to write this book but realized this insight is essential to the survival of many people.

I have found my patients and staff are great educators and indeed my patients help each other as much as I help them. These patients not only help their families and friends to understand their disease, but they also help others in allowing them to understand their own nerve problems.

It is certainly not my intention to make everyone who reads this book a physician, or those of us who are, better physicians. The job is not for everyone. What I do intend is those who are suffering can unlock their own innate capacity to understand their disease and heal themselves. The greatest gifts given to each of us are our own mind and good common sense. These have allowed people to evolve through the centuries, and it is my strong belief they will get us through the medical crisis we now face.

Pain

CHAPTER 1

"No pain, is dangerous
to our life and limb"

—Bernie Siegel, M.D.

This book is about people in pain. What many fail to understand is pain is a naturally occurring process in our bodies. As our body's way of letting us know something is wrong, it is a good and healthy warning sign. Certainly we understand when someone puts his or her hand down on a hot stove and removes it quickly, this is a good response. In this case, pain is letting us know there is an imminent danger and the body responds appropriately. It is only when we do not understand what the proper response is, or when this system goes awry, pain becomes a "problem."

This book is also about people getting rid of their pain. Although in many cases pain is caused by nerve problems, the theories, ideas, and techniques described in this book can be applied to pain from any origin. I have come to understand pain itself is defeatable. Further, within each of our minds lies the ability to control and even eliminate pain—safely, easily, and effectively.

1

"Susan" is a woman who came to me in pain. Her suffering was mental as well as physical, and as a result she was unable to keep up the pace of her regular job as an executive secretary for a highly successful corporate leader. Her job required extensive use of a computer and mouse as well as keying. Susan developed substantial problems with her hand, wrist, and arm and eventually a true cumulative trauma disorder. She had pain and discomfort all the way to her neck and significant problems with numbness, tingling, and severe pain and disability with her arm.

What became evident to both Susan and me was her job was the underlying cause of her pain. Although we tried her at extensive therapy along with modifications of the use of her arms on the computer, unfortunately she remained severely symptomatic. The issue came down to one of a choice, either losing the use of her limb or changing her career. We both suffered significantly with this decision. She became openly depressed at the thought of changing jobs or even limiting her hours. On the other hand, she had reached a point where she was unable to use her arm productively for any activities.

In this situation the doctor-patient relationship is vital. If I cannot find a reasonable avenue by which Susan can keep from worsening her own condition, I have failed at my mission. My solution must allow her to get rid of the pain and yet maintain her dignity and identity as a vital and successful human being. My job as a physician and healer is to teach my patients to adapt their lives and slow, halt, or reverse the disease processes.

Through the years as a surgeon dealing with my patients' pain, what has intrigued me more than anything is every individual's pain is perceived and tolerated differently. People have different pain levels in the face of the same disease, trauma, surgery, or pathology. It seems inconceivable that identical injuries and traumas can cause such drastically different reactions in different people, yet they do. Each of us has a nervous system that functions via the same biochemical principles, yet every individual responds differently to the same stimulus. Is this learned behavior or is it hereditary?

Pain is a teacher and, in fact, we need our pain. Anthony Robbins, author of *Unlimited Power*, points out pain is one of the great motivators for people to make change in their lives. He relates until a person has enough pain or suffers, there is insufficient motivation for him or her to move on or to try to improve or change the existing situation. Robbins describes a sequence of events that occurs prior to any major change in a person's life. The first is pain; the second is making a change or reacting to the pain when it becomes great enough. This leads to successive steps that ultimately result in successful relief of the pain and hopefully an improved life.

Robbins goes on to relate many of the great successes today that have occurred are due to people enduring enough pain or suffering to motivate them to take extreme measures.

Sometimes this takes a shock or an awakening event. I recall a lesson I learned many years ago when I was working as an undergraduate student in a rehabilitation center. The director was a wonderful and gentle man who was a quadriplegic. He had been involved in a car accident and was paralyzed from the neck down; he had truly known tragedy in his life. The circumstances surrounding this accident included the deaths of other members of his family. He was a strongly religious individual and only by his sheer faith and desire to help other people was he able to go on with his life.

There was a young patient speaking in his office, very much unaware of this doctor's situation. He went on for some time stating how his life was over because his lower leg had been amputated. He told of how the pain and discomfort he had gone through could not be understood by anyone. When he finished complaining, there was a stunned silence. He suddenly became aware of his doctor's paralysis. This rapidly put the young man's pain into perspective. He began to view his own very differently. Needless to say, this patient did well and went on to lead a normal life.

There is tremendous potential within the mind to eliminate or at least defer the impulses which are interpreted by the brain as pain. We have observed this with babies being delivered, legs amputated, and gall bladders removed while the patient is under hypnosis. Certainly, the stimuli are still there but somehow they never reach the brain's cortex to be interpreted. We have also seen how the very nature of the pain itself changes over the course of time. The mind actually reprograms its "circuits" to interpret what was once a painful stimulus as now a normal or sometimes even pleasant sensation.

A patient of mine, "Samantha," told me how after one of her hand surgeries the first thing she thought about was eating and getting her fingers moving. She said she "got a thrill out of the tingle." Every patient interprets dysesthesias or altered sensations differently. Many patients feel these normal postoperative symptoms of nerve burning and altered sensations and interpret them as painful or abnormal. Samantha, however, looked forward to this sensation because she knew right away the feeling meant everything was working. What a difference this attitude made! This patient experienced a positive result from her surgery and has done well. This attitudinal adjustment can be applied to pain from any source and enhances one's ability to deal with pain.

In *Love, Medicine and Miracles*, Dr. Bernie Siegel talks about medical miracles, miracle cures, and remissions. Indeed, I have seen many patients who had been told they would never be free of their disease who then went on to function normally. In fact, many achieved great feats acquiring new skills as well as resuming normal lives. I have seen patients heal their own nerves, turning their EMGs (nerve tests) from positive (abnormal) to negative (normal) and their pain into pleasure.

Only by experiencing these "miracles" firsthand and living through months and years together with these exceptional people have I come to appreciate this process. I am not a faith healer, but a surgeon. That along with the fact I was raised by a psychologist, has helped me formulate my own basic philosophies. In this book, I discuss real patients with physiologic disease and pain. I also address the innate human capacity everyone has to control, decrease, and even eliminate pain at its physiologic basis.

Early in her life, "Tara" attempted suicide after a personal tragedy. But she had a turnaround in her life and decided she would never quit anything or let anything ever again defeat her. Tara went from being suicidal to having four operations for nerve injury in as many years and brought herself to the status of a productive individual both as a mother and as a worker in society.

In *Think and Grow Rich*, author Napoleon Hill talks about burning desire as the one avenue by which people can attain riches both personally and financially. He describes this as an obsession whereby channeling all of one's positive mental and visceral emotions toward a defined goal almost invariably leads to success.

Hill relates a story about his own son who was born with no ears. It became obvious early on his son was deaf, and Hill was told by his son's physicians the child would never hear. Hill, practicing what he preached, told his son's doctors he would eventually hear as well as any other person. Blind faith, burning desire, and commitment were Hill's personal trademarks and what he preached for many years. He worked daily with his son for hours at a time trying to get him to respond to some stimuli. Ultimately, his son began to respond to auditory stimuli and eventually he developed the ability to hear. In fact, his son's hearing acuity was enough that he was able to communicate regularly. A hearing aid manufacturer heard about his son and made a special device for him which afforded, between his innate developed abilities and the hearing aid, full and complete ability to hear.

It is important to understand that pain and its relief often come from a burning desire to get better. Quite often obsession is the hallmark of miracle cures and exceptional patients. There is no doubt many patients succeed in healing themselves through their ability to shape this burning desire and move forward in spite of all odds appearing to be against them. I have found those patients who do have a burning desire to heal eventually find a way to rid themselves of their pain.

Perhaps we, as physicians, approach the treatment of our patients from the wrong direction. We continue to treat people by injecting them with poison and cutting them in the name of curing. We still sew people back together with needles and thread and operate with scalpels and scissors. We have blindly followed those who came before us.

This is our so-called modern medicine. Perhaps we have really missed the point and in our own egocentric way have convinced ourselves by removing the process from the person, we can cure the being. Instead, the true answer may be in allowing the person to cure himself or herself and keeping the doctor away long enough to allow the body to heal. When we graduate medical school, physicians take the hippocratic oath. One of the underlying tenents here is "primum non nosceri" (do no harm.) Perhaps we need to take a closer look at this statement. Looking back on those we have helped and those we have not, this becomes an even more startling reality.

I certainly don't claim to have all the answers but I do have many patients who got better after they had been told by others this was not possible. They improve not because I am a better doctor but because somehow deep inside I know my patients become better patients. They are allowed to be people and to take an active role in curing their own diseases. They take responsibility for their illness and for getting better. They understand there is no fault in failure but to not try is unforgivable!

"Beth," who worked as the driver of a large dump truck, had her fingers crushed when they were caught in the heavy steel trapdoor on the back of the truck. She had significant bone injury as well as nerve damage. Beth developed a severe pain syndrome in her arm secondary to her trauma. Beth has a strong work ethic and became severely depressed at her inability to continue working. She is a strong lady who is used to caring for herself, as well as caring for her family.

As if Beth had not endured enough pain, shortly after the accident, her daughter tragically was killed by an abusive ex-spouse. Beth experienced not only physical suffering but also the emotional devastation of self as well as family loss. She became severely depressed, exacerbating the underlying physical pain she already suffered. Refusing to succumb, Beth found a new path and used her pain to go forward. She took up the cause of protecting others like her daughter. She went from driving a truck to spearheading a national campaign to protect the rights of abused women. Beth is not rid of her pain and still has disability in her arm, but she has overcome this and moved on because of a burning desire to improve and become a leader rather than a victim. She turned multiple tragedy and personal pain into positive and productive activity.

I hope this book will give at least one person the insight and strength to pull himself or herself up out of the quagmire and get better in the face of a society that states too often there is "no cure." If this book helps only that one person to change his or her life from one of daily pain to one of pain free normal function, then it will have been well worth writing. As you read the following chapters, please remember this is not science fiction but rather a cumulative understanding of pain and our body's wonderful ability to deal with and actually eliminate the devastating impact of disease. There is an answer to every problem; the key is just in knowing where and how to look for it. More often than not, looking for answers within is much more effective than looking without.

Healing— Who Can Do It?

CHAPTER 2

"So long as a man imagines
that he cannot do this or that,
so long is he determined not to do it:
and consequently,
so long it is impossible to him
that he should do it."

—Benedict (Baruch) Spinoza

Healing is a basic part of our nature and physiology. Animals of all species, at all levels, have the capacity to heal themselves. We homo sapiens are the only species that have formalized this into the complex system we call medical care. Many animals care for and nurture their ill and lick their own wounds but almost all heal the same way. Bones heal by forming new bone. Nerves and all other structures heal by forming scar tissue. The nature of this healing process is quite sophisticated yet simple. Basically the body forms scar to take the place of the injured tissue. Given the proper time, environment, and tender loving care, most injuries do heal, and rather well!

9

We know the more aggressively and poorly we treat scar tissue, the more a malignant or "bad" scar is formed. A good example is a scab that is picked or rubbed with salt every day. This will form a significant keloid or large ugly scar. By contrast, one treated with a bandage and salve and left alone tends to heal very cosmetically.

"Tony" has worked for the postal service for some time. Because of his work responsibilities there, Tony developed severe tendinitis and needed surgery on his right hand. He had severe scarring internally around the tendon structures and nerves. In spite of extensive conservative treatment, Tony has continued to exacerbate his pain and symptoms with aggressive activities. Tony required surgery at one point for his left shoulder. The scar that formed afterward was a large, ugly keloid. He subsequently returned to work but has had progressive problems with inflammation, pain, and scarring in his arms.

Tony forms very heavy scars. Operations and aggressive insults (that is, heavy work) to his arms result in inflammation and swelling beyond what is experienced in the general population. Based on this knowledge, the key to Tony's healing process has been conservative care and lifestyle modification. He's been taken away from the heavy grabbing, repetitive, and lifting activities he performed while working. This has helped to calm down his symptoms. In fact, Tony is still in the process of modifying his lifestyle. He is an individual with a very strong will and is moving slowing but steadily in a healing direction. The key to helping Tony heal is not my being a surgeon but rather my being an educator. The more Tony understands his disease and decreases the repeated insults to his body, the better his chances are of healing. If, however, I am not successful in re-educating him, Tony will no doubt go on to further problems and progressive long-term disability. He is currently exploring a return to school and a major career change. He is in control of his future and of his pain.

The healing process is very straightforward in humans. When nerves and structures are injured, scar tissue forms and takes the shape and place of the normal tissue. This tissue forms in definite stages and over definite periods of time. I like to term "scar formation" as either good or bad scar. Good scar is scar that forms in a similar nature, look, feel, and, if dissected, microscopic appearance, to the tissue it is replacing. It is fine tissue that forms very much like a cobweb, structurally beautiful—its manner and function much like the tissue it is repairing and/or replacing. Unfortunately, when scar malforms in a dissimilar way, it creates what I term "bad scar." This creates a thick, ugly tenacious scar. Instead of allowing good function, it inhibits and, in fact, stands in its way. This bad scar is the culprit in many nerve and orthopaedic problems. Ultimately, this is what renders the individual disabled by inhibiting normal function.

The key factor here is we all have within us the capacity to heal ourselves and get rid of our pain. If we just *allow* our bodies to heal, most problems do get better. This process may be short or long (sometimes extending to months and years), but it is predictable. This is a definable pattern and as long as we can follow this pattern and understand it, almost all of us heal.

When we look at nerves and nerve injury, the healing process is essentially no different. When nerves are cut, there is an actual degeneration of the nerve fibers within the sheath. Essentially the dendrite portion of the nerve dies and the sheath itself remains. Over the course of time, a new nerve regenerates or grows through this sheath. If the sheath is surgically repaired or only partially cut, the nerve can find the other side and grow through (regenerate).

A similar process occurs when nerves are injured, except the regeneration process is less hindered by severe scarring.

"Sophia" is a young woman who went to New York to study and become an actress. Unfortunately, she didn't study bagel cutting and sustained a bagel slicing injury. She went through the bagel and into her hand with the point of a knife. (This is a common injury, and I highly recommend extreme caution when slicing bagels. A similar injury occurs when trying to separate frozen hamburgers with a sharp knife. Invariably, many people do get the point (and I mean this literally.) Sophia sustained an injury to one of the nerves in her index finger. She was told when she was sewn up in the emergency room surgery would be required to repair the nerve. When I evaluated her, I noted there was some intact low-level function (that is, she had some feeling but mostly pain). We opted to take the conservative route rather than surgery, and she has had excellent return of function. Sensation is coming back to normal and there is regeneration without the need for an open surgical repair. This is consistent with a partial cut of the nerve and the fact that there was enough fiber still intact to allow regeneration and regrowth of the nerve through the sheath.

The ultimate example of regeneration is the starfish, which will actually regrow its own limb when amputated. If you believe in evolution (and as a scientist, I do), then indeed at some time we all had this capacity somewhere in our genes. Perhaps some day we will understand this better and be able to more completely heal patients by unlocking this process.

A local physician who is a naturopath became a patient of mine when he attempted to repair a garage door and amputated his finger. "Dave" had a successful replant of his digit when we performed his surgery but had a severe fracture through his distal phalanx (the bone at the tip of the finger). This was, by its very nature, a difficult fracture to heal. In spite of our best surgical efforts, we were not able to get the two ends of the bone close enough to heal easily. Normally, fancy devices, including one called a bone stimulator, are used to get these injuries to heal. The bone stimulator helps fracture healing by electrically stimulating the osteoblasts (the bone-forming cells) to do their job a bit more efficiently and aggressively. In many cases, this is not successful and further surgery is necessary to actually add extra bone to obtain healing. Dave, being the dynamic individual he is and a naturopath by training, told me he just used a magnet, placing this over the fracture a few times a day. I cannot tell you whether it was his magnet or Dave's own personal magnetism but this fracture healed faster and more solidly than any fracture of its kind I have ever treated. Further, his digit has done better than most and I attribute this all to his positive attitude and personal experiences with the body's ability to heal itself. Given the proper frame of mind and treatment, people heal and heal well.

It is well documented that chemical messengers in the body called endorphins and enkephalins are released by happy and positive thoughts. These enhance the body's natural healing process. Nerves tend to function better in a wholesome environment. Nourishment from a good diet, rest, improved breathing and circulation, and increased blood supply help nerves heal better. When injured nerves are treated well, the new scar "beds," which form around the scar, are also more conducive to good nerve healing.

Conversely, an individual who does not get enough rest, does not eat well, gets no exercise, and has an overall low level of endorphin and enkephalins not only heals poorly but also heals less completely. The function of these poorly healed nerves is often, as you now understand, severely compromised. This can result in long-term chronic pain and dysfunction.

"Ben" is a truck driver who came to us after sustaining a severe injury to the nerves of his brachial plexus, which are all the nerves that travel from the neck to the arm between the neck and shoulder. Because of his injury, he was unable to perform any normal activities with his arm or do his job, which consisted of driving a truck and lifting up to 200 pounds. Electromyleogram (EMG)/Nerve conduction studies (NCV) demonstrated severely positive findings indicating actual nerve damage.

Ben undertook our program with the attitude he was going to get better and go back to what he was doing. I told him from the beginning very few people with a similar injury actually return to that level of function, but he assured me he would heal to this extent. I did not discourage him but still maintained a certain amount of reservation. To my surprise and delight, Ben taught me an invaluable lesson. Not only did he heal, but his subsequent EMG/NCV testing showed he had actually reversed the damage in his nerves and healed these completely. His objective nerve tests showed his nerves were normal. He is now back to truck driving and performing heavy duty work in spite of all the odds and statistics. This is not a person I cured but rather a person who cured himself with an excellent attitude and vision. He visualized himself back at his job performing his regular activities and indeed achieved this because of his willingness to meet the challenge and take it on with vigor.

I often advise my patients to modify their lifestyle to live within the limits of their disease. This is important. It does *not* mean lying down and doing nothing. Conversely, it means simply not doing activities that aggravate their pain! Eliminating pain is no different than any other healing, be it scar tissue or bone. Healing takes place as part of the body's natural mechanism. It is the norm and can be expected to happen. We simply need to *allow* the body to pursue its own natural course and healing will follow.

You will find there is a basic theme regarding pain management. If the patient can grasp this and understand it, then he will have achieved something and likely will heal. Pain does burn out and goes away most of the time. Given the proper time, care, knowledge, and desire, any individual can defeat his or her pain.

Faith Healing Versus Faith in Healing

CHAPTER 3

*"The physician's method of delivering truth
to the patient can help combat or help
intensify disease. If delivered in the wrong
way, the truth can produce pain and
erode hope—a dismal state that hardly offers
an ideal environment for making the most
of the physician's ministrations.
If delivered the right way, however, the truth
can bolster the patient's will to live and
various plus factors can come into play."*

—Norman Cousins

We all have within us the ability to heal. Basically, all we need is some help to bring this out. Very often, this simply requires either finding someone who cares or caring enough about ourselves to do it. It means we have enough faith in ourselves to allow utilization of this capacity. Many times educating my patients about their disease becomes the one significant factor in allowing self-healing.

Linda is a woman who is a survivor. She has been an insulin dependent diabetic since childhood and lived with all of the issues that go along with diabetes including many of the myths.

Linda has taken the time to thoroughly understand her disease. She knows that diabetes is a disease of the micro-circulation and when this is well controlled diabetics can lead normal lives.

Aside from being a mother, Linda chose a career as a certified nurse assistant in which she used her arms aggressively. During the course of her work, Linda sustained a significant injury to her arm when a large patient lost her balance. As the patient fell, she grabbed and yanked Linda's arm. Unfortunately, this caused a yanking or tractioning injury to the nerves of the brachial plexus at the level of the thoracic outlet between the neck and shoulder. She had severe unrelenting pain in her entire extremity.

Linda was told that all of her symptoms were related to her diabetes and not the injury. She was further told that because of her diabetes she was not a candidate for surgical intervention and would never get better. Thankfully her family physician recognized her significant nerve injury and sent her in for further evaluation.

Linda and I had extensive discussions on multiple occasions concerning options for her conservative as well as operative care. She failed to improve after extensive therapy and ultimately did request surgical intervention. Linda has since had three surgeries.

Her first surgery at the carpal tunnel went well. She received wonderful relief at the hand and wrist but not at the thoracic outlet. She basically "proved the critics wrong" by improving after this surgery.

Her second surgery was on the ulnar nerve at the elbow. She did not have as easy a time with this surgery as the first. In fact, Linda continued with significant pain and discomfort after the surgery. This was due to a severe nerve injury and scarring at the third level or thoracic outlet.

We were able to stabilize the significant exacerbation of her pain with therapy, and Linda continued to work at regaining her elbow and arm motion. She remained astutely aware that her major problem was at the thoracic outlet level and her lower arm symptoms were secondary issues. We were able to push forward because of Linda's persistence, faith, and understanding of her disease. She recovered from her second surgery and ultimately did have surgery at the level of the thoracic outlet (a dangerous but often rewarding surgery).

When Linda awoke from her thoracic outlet surgery, she told me that although she had faith in me, she was now certain she was right. Not only was her major problem in the thoracic outlet, but also her diabetes was not a factor. Her pain was gone!

Although diabetics may be somewhat predisposed to develop peripheral nerve problems (i.e. carpal tunnel) when their disease is poorly controlled, this is often not the underlying cause. Linda had a classic traction injury to the nerves of her brachial plexus and was certain that her diabetes was not the cause of her pain. A "peripheral neuropathy" was not the issue.

Linda understood that she had severe nerve scarring and entrapment due to an injury and not her diabetes. This was consistent with the scar tissue we found at surgery which, when released, gave her relief from her symptomotology.

Linda's ability to overcome her severe debilitating injury was marked by a combination of a trusting relationship between patient and physician and sheer will and determination. She has been an inspiration to me and my staff as a survivor who successfully fought an uphill battle against the system as well as against her disease.

Dr. Bernie Siegel points to a theory in his book *Peace, Love, and Healing* to explain why cancer develops in certain individuals with a depressed immune system (the body's defense system against disease). He explains that the immune and nervous systems are interrelated. Indeed, they control each other. He also brings out the fact that stress results in an alteration of the immune system's function in the body. This stress can compromise the immune system resulting in cancer or, in the case of the nervous system, dysfunction. When the nervous system is functioning abnormally, pain is a very probable and often real manifestation.

It is known that with stress, the white blood cell count in the body will increase. This can be physical stress following, for example, surgery or emotional stress at a time of grief or anxiety. The key factor to understand here is that the nervous system itself, when strongly stimulated, influences other physiologic processes in the body. It becomes quite apparent that a depressed nervous system will depress our other body systems and compromise healing processes and normal functions.

Faith healing and faith healers have survived many centuries. Many so-called miracles have been attributed to magic potions, medicines, medicine men, and religion. It is interesting to me that, although I strongly believe in God, I can attribute many miracles to people. It is the miracles that occur *within* individuals and not to individuals I find most fascinating. How many stories have we all heard about people performing superhuman feats such as mothers lifting cars off a child and people who have been told they would never walk again who get up and actually run? Are these miracles or strictly acts of unflappable faith? We all know if we try and try and try again, we will generally succeed in performing a task or learning a specific art form or behavior. Surely, we all have our own innate talents, but we all have the ability to live, learn, love, have fun, and heal! To succeed is simply a matter of believing we can and having the inner strength to try—the-little-engine-that-could syndrome.

Tara is the woman previously mentioned who attempted suicide early in life. She related to me in a visit that after the suicide episode, she crystallized many of her ideas and had a turnaround in her life. She decided at that point she would never quit anything again and never let anything defeat her. Tara has had a number of surgeries on her arm and at one point improved enough to be able to go back into training and the working world. When she graduated from a school which specialized in people with handicaps, she wrote the following:

Life Changes in a Minute

Sometime after 8:00 P.M. on July 10, 1989, my life changed forever. I thought I had it made for life. Working as a packager was the kind of job I liked to do. I liked the work. I liked the people. I especially liked the money. In one split second, one movement of my right arm it was over. The next few years were filled with physical therapy, surgery, a lot of pain, and depression. After three months of physical therapy, surgery was tried. The operation was successful; but as dedicated as I am, I talked the doctor into letting me return to work. What a mistake! I worked part-time for six weeks and the surgery was ruined. It took two more operations and years of physical therapy just to be able to use my arm and hand again. The pain was excruciating at times. Many days, I didn't want to get out of bed; I didn't think I could make it. Those times were especially rough for my daughter, Jeannie, who remembered what I was like before the injury. But I'm a survivor! My famous saying to everyone no matter how down I got was "I'll survive." I guess, if you say it often enough, you begin to believe it. Here is a poem a friend gave to me that helped me make it through the most depressing times.

Don't Quit

When things go wrong as they sometimes will
When the road you're trudging seems all up hill
When the funds are low and the debts are high
And you want to smile, but you have to sigh
When care is pressing you down a bit
Rest, if you must, but don't you quit.

Life is queer with its twists and turns,
As everyone of us sometimes learns,
And many a failure turns about
When he might have won had he stuck it out:
Don't give up though the pace seems slow
You may succeed with another blow.
Success is failure turned inside out
The silver tint of the clouds of doubt
And you never can tell how close you are,
It may be near when it seems so far;
So stick to the fight when you're hardest hit
It's when things seem worst that you must not quit.

This poem really helped me to see things differently. I began working in my garden again, took long walks at Valley Forge, and was blessed with a new daughter (Suzie) in March, 1992. I finally admitted to myself that I couldn't return to my job. In September when I came to The Disabled Persons Work Reentry Program, it was a new beginning to my life. My outlook for the future is good. I'm doing well and I can't wait to see where the road leads.

Tara has undergone brachial plexus surgery since this writing. This is major surgery generally requiring six months of recovery time. She was in for her four-week postoperative visit and had done so well she was out in her garden working on her roses and returned to work at her job with an engineering firm. She is a wonderful example of a person who understood believing in herself and understanding her own disease are generally enough to march forward against all odds and win.

The ultimate capacity of this inner strength is generally unknown to each of us. Only in times of great trial and challenge do we discover our true capabilities. Sometimes it is just a matter of finding the right motivation or path. At other times, it is being placed in a situation where there simply is no choice. The key here is that faith in one's own ability to heal is essential in any healing process.

It is unfortunate we cannot retain this innate capacity from childhood. Survival and learning are instinctive. Those parents reading this are also well aware that children are willing to try anything. It seems age and maturity are often not good mentors for survival.

This brings to mind "Joe," a dynamic young man who has been through significant emotional as well as physical pain from his injury. He is a fighter who has outstanding support from his wife and family. He faces his injury with the attitude he is going to go forward and live his life normally. What Joe doesn't realize is he has been a tremendous positive influence on the other patients around him.

One day I was in our therapy unit making my rounds as I normally do seeing my post-op patients. (I like to see them in therapy because it gives me a chance to see what's really going on. I hear people tell their therapists more than they tell their docs!) Joe was post-op from the first stage of a reconstructive procedure; in an industrial accident he had lost all the fingers on his hand except his thumb. We had placed an artificial tendon in his thumb in hope of at least giving him some function in the way of grasp.

As I was evaluating a young woman sitting next to Joe, he asked her what she had done. She said, "My carpal tunnel and it feels great." He paused for a second, looked at her, then at me and said with a twinkle in his eye, "Boy, you are lucky. When I went into surgery, I thought I was just having my carpal tunnel done too. Look what happened to my hand." There was of course a flurry of laughter throughout the unit. One could just sense the healing effect this had not only on Joe himself but on all the other individuals around him.

This man is a credit to himself as well as an example of the concept of attitude making healing occur. He continues to progress well with respect to both his life and his hand.

Another patient, "Jack," and I had a discussion one day about his abilities to undertake treatment and go along with it. He told me he thought I was a wonderful doctor and that my seat was the most difficult one to be in. I told Jack I felt just the opposite; his was indeed the toughest seat. He gave me the following advice, which I have not only shared with my other patients but also applied to my own life.

Jack told me when he undertakes any venture, business or personal, he investigates the people he is working with thoroughly. He does a complete research on background and gets as much information as he can about them. He finds the person he feels knows the most about that area, more than he ever could hope to know. He then contracts with that person to undertake the job or, in the case of medical treatment, his care. At that point he is able to relax, confident he can simply follow the advice given to him. It is important to understand this is *not* passive patient participation but active. He actively seeks the people he feels most confident with and then shares control with someone who he feels has the ability to make decisions he cannot.

Jack follows my advice, though he often questions and "alters" my suggestions. This is a man who has found a wonderful way to meld his own personal healing abilities with my instructive and surgical capabilities. Indeed between the two of us he has made excellent progress and attained good relief from his nerve problems.

I have also noted significant differences in patients' outcomes from surgery simply by things said while they are sedated or asleep in the operating room. There have been rare instances over the years where, due to events beyond my control, I was not able to say "good night" to a patient before they went under anesthesia for an operation. I like to do this to let the patient know I am there and we are "in it together" as partners in the healing process. There is no doubt; these patients did not do as well post-operatively. They were somewhat more depressed and delayed in their healing processes.

Dr. Siegel points out in his writings the efficacy of the power of suggestion to patients under anesthesia. He relates episodes of patients stopping their own bleeding during surgery. He also emphasizes the wonderful soothing effects of music. This effect has been well documented in recent studies not only for the patient but in helping the surgeon perform his job better as well.

I had a confirmatory experience not too long ago when I was operating on a patient and was feeling particularly calm and relaxed. I did not understand my unusual sense of ease that day. We didn't even have a radio in the room and I couldn't listen to music as I almost always do. Suddenly as I was completing the operation, I became aware of harp music wafting gently throughout the entire operative corridor. It was only then I realized "Maria," a music therapist and an extraordinary harpist, was playing for my next patient in the preoperative. She was playing to prepare "Lori" mentally for her surgery. She was also helping prepare me to handle my day and my surgeries better as well. I now have some tape recordings of Maria's music, and I use them to prepare myself and my patients for surgery.

It has been my experience that patients who know someone is there who cares for them have much better outcomes. The people who care mean everyone from doctors and nurses to family and friends. There are fewer side effects from anesthesia and less postoperative pain when people simply know they are loved.

We have noted the mind's extraordinary ability to control physiologic responses. As you will learn later, I do a tremendous amount of work with biofeedback techniques and deep-breathing exercises. Via these techniques, patients can often control and sometimes eliminate pain and discomfort. These have also been used to treat patients with blood pressure problems. Many of my patients' operations are performed under what we call local anesthesia with sedation. This type of anesthesia allows the patient to be in a semi-awake state and not risk undergoing general anesthesia where they are fully asleep.

On one particular day, my patient's blood pressure rose to 200/130 during an operation under local anesthesia. (This sometimes happens because of the stress of surgery). When his pressure got this high, he was actually in danger of having a stroke. We had to consider stopping the operation at this point. "Ralph" had gone through our biofeedback training program so I decided to try something.

I turned to him and said, "Ralph, I need you to use your biofeedback techniques and bring your blood pressure down. This will allow me to continue your surgery." He responded immediately by doing his exercises and his pressure went down to normal. I was able to successfully complete the operation and, in fact, we needed less anesthesia for sedation and pain control. He was able to tolerate the surgery without any further event. I am certain his ability to utilize his own mind to control his pain and his faith in our relationship are what got him through that surgery.

It has been my experience patients can control their own nervous system responses and pain if they are simply taught how. This is widely accepted in the way of hypnotic suggestion and pain management. Pain has been controlled using hypnosis for many years. I don't know why our medical community has not yet accepted these concepts and taken them even further. We doctors need to have more faith in our patients rather than asking our patients to have more faith in us. When I listen closely, my patients tell me exactly what is wrong—and often how to fix it!

My advice to all potential patients is to find someone who cares and use this person. If someone believes in you and allows you to believe in yourself and your abilities, you can often heal yourself.

Unfortunately, the opposite holds true as well. It has occurred to me we may be approaching medicine from a completely antiquated point of view. Perhaps the concept perpetuated over time that doctors are healers is in error. Could it be the patients are the healers and doctors should just augment this process? Surgeons are certainly good as technicians and, with properly timed procedures, can be helpful in the overall treatment plan. The healing though really needs to come from within the patient.

I wonder if we have really come that far. Indeed the days of leeches being used for medicinal purposes are back. Leeches are being used again to help in replanted (replaced) digits. When the digits become congested, leeches help to drain the venous blood. I often ask myself, have we really progressed or simply come full circle?

Another problem in our society is we, as patients, often have unrealistic expectations. Almost daily, someone comes into my office and says to me, "Doctor, make me better" or "Fix me." My answer is always indeed I am here to help and if they need surgery, I will perform this for them. I also tell them the only one who can really get them better is themselves. When I speak to these people further, it is apparent many are still looking for the so-called 1990s cure: take a pill, have an operation, and off you go. The fact is things do not always go that way. Patients sometimes get worse rather than better after surgery, and we, as a medical community, do not discuss this with our

27

patients often enough. We don't prepare them or ourselves. We allow these unrealistic expectations to continue and only after a catastrophe or the patient is in real trouble do we then allow them to make choices.

Patients must learn to take responsibility for their illness and *from day one* understand the decisions made are not only ours, as physicians, but theirs as well. We may empathize with our patients and their outcomes, but our patients live with their disease and pain every minute of every day. Results, good or bad, are *their* reality and become part of *their* lives.

Physicians and healers must be aware that people today do have the capacity to understand their disease. Our job is to educate our patients so they can make intelligent decisions concerning their own illness and govern their treatment. I tell my patients it is not I who will decide if and when they need an operation but rather they who will tell me. It is a rare circumstance when my patient does not know better than I when and what type of operation he or she may need.

A prime example of this today is carpal tunnel syndrome. Indeed carpal tunnel syndrome has become very commonly diagnosed for a number of reasons. Initially, carpal tunnel was a disease mainly found in elderly ladies who knitted or crocheted too much. They had classic symptoms of night pain, numbness, and tingling. This responded very well to a conservative, relatively straightforward operation. Simply releasing the ligament in this sedentary, elderly population gave enough relief. These patients had very low demand on their hands.

Unfortunately, this diagnosis is not sufficient to address many of today's nerve problems. Some are carpal tunnel but others are more complex problems.

"Steve" is a young man who has been through a lot in his life. Our first encounter was at 4:00 A.M. in the emergency room after he had crushed his left hand. He was accompanied by his wife and they asked me before anything else, "Are you the best there is?" I told them I was not but there weren't a lot of people up and about at 4:00 A.M. Steve and I quickly developed a good relationship, and we spent the next few weeks trying to salvage as much of his hand as we could. He underwent a number of surgeries including placement of artificial tendons and treatment of broken bones and injured nerves and blood vessels in his hand. He subsequently lost his fifth digit, but we were able to save the rest of his hand.

The nature of Steve's injuries was such that he had significant involvement not only of the tendons, bones, and muscles in the hand but also of the nerves in the hand and arm. He later required thoracic outlet surgery as well as surgery to free his median nerve at the wrist and hand at the level of the carpal tunnel.

Throughout the seven years I've known Steve, he has lived with daily pain. He has, however, remained an optimistic and happy individual. During the course of Steve's comeback, he endured a significant amount of physical as well as mental punishment. He set himself back a number of times. In spite of all this, Steve's outlook generally remains optimistic and although he lives daily with pain, he continues to move forward and enjoy life. Steve's basic attitude is if he keeps on going, he'll always be ahead of the game. He has taught me a lot about working through injuries and pain. He is a wonderful example of someone whose faith in himself, combined with an understanding of his long-term goals, has allowed him to keep on going instead of just lying down and becoming a statistic.

The unfortunate reality is many patients today who complain of numbness are simply labeled and categorized as having "carpal tunnel syndrome." Consequently, the diagnosis and treatment plan falters. There is a tremendous misconception among many practitioners as well as those involved from a corporate point of view that "all that is numb is carpal tunnel and if it is not carpal tunnel, you must be crazy." There are many good doctors who treat nerve problems but confusion and problems often ensue, unless the patient fits the standard carpal tunnel picture.

It has become vitally important for patients to understand their disease and help their physicians understand the pathophysiology of their specific problems. Many people who come to me with this diagnosis (carpal tunnel) do not end up in surgery. They modify their lives and learn to live within the limitations of their disease—just as our patients who have surgery.

Many patients have surgery and do not get better (up to 20 percent in the literature today). This is due in part to the presence of significant disease and in part to poor communication and understanding between patient and doctor. Many actually become worse because they continue to be exposed to the environment and hazards that brought them to our offices in the first place—they return to the workplace that caused the problem instead of understanding this return is fraught with danger of recurrence, or worse!

Carpal Tunnel— What Is It?

CHAPTER 4

Carpal tunnel problems are diagnosed in millions of Americans every year. This may well be the single most commonly operated problem in American society today. Recent statistics indicate there are approximately a half million carpal tunnel surgeries performed annually in the United States. The economic cost of these procedures is in excess of 2 billion dollars. It may well also be the single most overoperated diagnosis today as well. Somewhere between 10 and 20 percent of these patients have either recurrent problems or continued problems after the surgery.

Carpal tunnel is reported to have a prevalence of between one and 10 percent in the general population. It is much higher in specific occupational groups, ranging from 17.1 to 61.5 percent of workers. It is found more commonly in people who perform repetitive activities such as bankers, sanders, grocery store workers, factory workers, secretaries, computer workers, and the like.

"Sarah" came to me while she was working as a checker in a supermarket. She performed repeated activities with her hands and arms in the way of scanning and punching in pricing codes to the register. She developed significant problems with numbness and tingling in her hands and arms. She became symptomatic to the point where she was not able to function well and was concerned about the significant progression of her symptoms. Luckily she came to see me early on.

We were able to remove Sarah from her offending environment and avoid the need for any surgery. With therapy and lifestyle modification, she went on to lead a normal life. She is expecting her second child and having no difficulties with her hands and arms. In fact, she is now a travel agent and doing very well because of her astute recognition of her significant problem and institution of early conservative care.

Many times the diagnosis of carpal tunnel problems is either incorrect or incomplete. Many of these people have substantially different problems than the disease that is "diagnosed." Some patients are also sent back to the same job or same type of jobs and activities that caused their problem in the first place. When they continue to have problems and symptoms they are told, "you had the operation and you are just going to have to live with these symptoms and the pain." They are told they need to accept their continued symptomatology as just another part of their lives.

Many of these patients never return to their previous jobs and never get relief or complete relief from their symptoms. In fact, it has been stated carpal tunnel problems have reached "epidemic proportions" in the United States today. The problem extends much further than simple discomfort or pain while working. Many people I see are not able to function with respect to taking care of their children and/or spouses. This is a far-reaching issue with many ramifications, especially when treated inappropriately or left to go on without complete diagnosis or treatment.

Carpal Tunnel Syndrome

In the early 1950s, Dr. G.S. Phalen described a syndrome in which patients had numbness, tingling, and at times pain and discomfort in the hand and specifically in the thumb, index, and long fingers. In some, the pain radiated up to the arm and neck. Night pain often awakened these patients. Activities such as crocheting or needlepoint aggravated the condition. The symptom complex popularly became known as carpal tunnel syndrome. I must openly admit I miss the days when I saw people who simply had straightforward simple "carpal tunnel problems." Although some patients still fall into this category, today they are the exception rather than the rule.

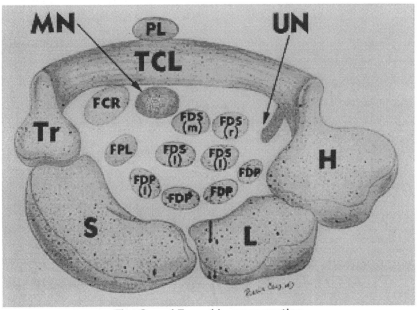

The Carpal Tunnel in cross section
TCL: Transverse Carpal Ligament; MN: Median nerve; T.R., S, L, H: Carpal bones; FDS, FDP, etc: Flexor Tendons

Anatomically, the carpal tunnel as pictured consists of a closed space bound on the volar or the palm side of the hand by a ligament called the transverse carpal ligament. This attaches to four bones of the wrist joint and forms the roof of the carpal canal. The other bones of the wrist form the deep part or the floor of the carpal canal. Through the tunnel travel the flexor tendons, which are the cables that move our fingers. These allow us to make a fist and these tendons glide approximately one and one-half inches up and down the arm. They are controlled by muscles and allow us to make a fist by pulling our digits down. The median nerve lies on the palm side of these tendons directly above and sits directly below the ligament.

It is important to understand these structures are not small but rather substantial, good-sized units that can be physically manipulated. Each of these tendons is approximately the size of a thick piece of linguine. They are equally as smooth and slippery. The median nerve itself is about the size of a pencil and again is a rather smooth structure. Each of these can be easily identified within the carpal tunnel, and it is important to realize these are structures we can see, feel, touch, and hold in understanding how treatment from a surgical point of view can occur.

I must confess when I was in medical school and studied nerves, tendons, and blood vessels, the nerves always evaded me as a nondescript entity. I thought of them as imaginary structures we could not really see but yet touched every cell and millimeter of the body. It appeared to me a magical phenomenon that something could actually make us feel, move, and function.

I later discovered not only are they real, but they are also substantial in nature. Over the course of years, I have come to realize, although they do indeed function magically, their destinations are predictable and relatively easily traced. After having the opportunity to touch, feel, hold, and even repair many of these structures, both under direct vision as well as with a microscope, there is little magic. Although we don't know exactly how nerves work, we do know what they look like and that they are predictable in their response to trauma, compression, and stretch.

The median nerve was Helen Keller's window to the world. She had no ability to see or hear and communicated with the

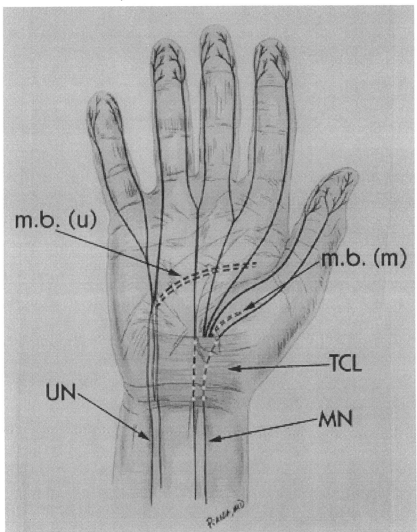

m.b. (u)

m.b. (m)

TCL

UN

MN

The median nerve at the wrist travels through the carpal tunnel beneath the transverse carpal ligament (TCL). The Ulnar Nerve has its own separate tunnel (the Canal of Guyon). [m.b. (m): motor branch median nerve; m.b. (u): motor branch ulnar nerve; UN: ulnar nerve; MN: median nerve] world through touch. What was most important to Helen Keller was her ability to feel things. The ability to read Braille as well as most of the sensory input from feel in the hand comes through the median nerve. In essence, the median nerve was Helen Keller's eyes, and as anyone who has read her work will attest, it gave her a tremendous view of the world. In fact, through her median nerve, Helen Keller observed more than most of us who have sight and hearing.

The underlying mechanism of carpal tunnel problems is inflammation within this closed tunnel at the wrist. The tendons that glide through the carpal tunnel are surrounded and encased in a lining called tenosynovium. This is a very thin, filmy substance responsible for making these tendons slippery and allowing them to glide easily through the carpal tunnel. When the fingers are moved rapidly and regularly or the wrist is bent up and down (flexed and extended), the tenosynovium may heat up or become swollen. This results from simple friction. It is no different than rubbing our hands together or rubbing two sticks together: The end result is heat. When the tenosynovium heats up, it becomes somewhat swollen and mildly increases in its space-occupying qualities. If enough swelling occurs and the synovium becomes thick enough, this will take up more space in the carpal tunnel. Because the carpal tunnel is closed on all sides, this eventually will put increased pressure on all the structures within, including the median nerve. This increase in pressure results in the production of nerve symptoms such as numbness and tingling and, at times, pain and discomfort.

I had an experience when I was an intern that reinforced this concept of swelling and inflammation and the production of nerve symptoms. I received a call from one of the floor nurses at about 2:00 A.M. who thought I should take a look at a patient's arm. She related the patient was complaining of numbness and tingling in her hand. Apparently someone had started an intravenous line (a small catheter inserted into the arm to give patients fluid). When this is done, a tourniquet or tight band is placed on the upper arm and this allows the veins to be seen more easily. Unfortunately, the line was placed but the tourniquet was never taken off the arm. Approximately 2 liters of fluid were run into the arm by a pump. The fluid could not go past the tourniquet, therefore, it filled the arm, forearm, and carpal tunnel.

When I arrived on the floor, I met an elderly lady who was not completely oriented but was aware enough to know her hand and arm felt different. I took a complete history and then examined the patient. Even as an intern, it did not take me long to surmise the nature of the problem. I will never forget the scene when we opened this patient's hand and about a gallon of water came gushing out of the carpal canal. It certainly was overemphasis of a point but did indeed prove increased fluid and swelling in the carpal canal will result in the predicted nerve symptoms. They also resolved once the pressure was released.

As you may recall, the median nerve supplies feeling to the thumb, index, long, and thumb side of the ring or fourth finger. This is the classic description of the distribution of the nerve symptoms although any one finger or all of these may be affected. Patients will at times also complain of symptoms with discomfort radiating to the upper arm or neck level. There are various theories as to what actually happens to cause the nerve to become symptomatic, but suffice it to say at this point the actual blood supply and circulation to the nerve and its ability to function normally are hampered.

What I have just described is an early stage of carpal tunnel problems. It is obvious most of us do not continue to move our hand and wrist 24 hours a day and the traumas or insults to the nerve are usually intermittent. What occurs over the course of time is that this swelling or tendinitis reveals itself whenever the structures in the carpal canal are subject to injury, be it in the way of direct trauma such as hitting our hands on the wheel of the car in a motor vehicle accident or with constant stress activities such as repetitive motion or regular motion. When the swelling puts enough pressure on the nerve, the surrounding sheath of the nerve or the mesoepineurium itself becomes inflamed.

Over the course of time, where there is swelling in the carpal tunnel with inflammation about the tendons (tenosynovitis) and pressure on the nerve, causing further swelling of the surrounding mesoepineurium, a cyclical situation occurs. Eventually as the swelling increases and then decreases throughout the course of a day or work week, a congealing of the inflamed tissue ensues. Ultimately, this results in the formation of pathologic scar tissue surrounding the nerve as well as the tendons. This scar tissue normally looks very much like a cobweb. When pathologic, it looks more like someone poured glue around the nerve, binding it severely, rather than gently holding it in place. The scarring prevents the nerve from gliding or sliding through the tissues as it normally does. If the nerve cannot move well and is bound down, two conditions occur. The first is a direct constriction or essentially strangling of the nerve resulting in nerve symptoms on a more regular basis. The second is the nerve is now more compromised and it takes less swelling or pressure to produce nerve symptoms.

Ultimately, the nerve may become fixed to the point where reaching overhead or bending and posturing of the wrist cause a pulling or tractioning on the nerve-reproducing symptoms by simply changing positions of the wrist or arm. This becomes a secondary issue independent of the tendinitis and at this point we have a fixed nerve problem. If this is allowed to go on to very late stages, that is, continuing to key at a computer or scan at the checkout, the nerve can actually cease to function properly and begin to die. At this point, numbness becomes a permanent fixture and muscle wasting may occur. The thenar muscles may begin to waste and die. These are the muscles at the base of the thumb in the palm and are very important in that they allow palmar abduction or opposition of the thumb. The opposable thumb allows us to write and grasp tools. The opposable thumb is basically what distinguishes man's manipulations from the ape. It allows us to pick up a quarter off the floor, to write, or to pinch a baby's cheek. The opposable thumb has allowed homo sapiens to advance beyond the ape and many feel this a most important factor in the evolution of man. Certainly the stage of wasting and permanent numbness is a very late stage and occurs only in severe cases neglected or untreated for many years.

"Jane" came to me after many years of working at repetitive activities at a manufacturing plant. She had severe problems with pain, numbness, and tingling in her hands and had reached a point where she had complete loss of sensation. The pain and discomfort were so bad she was unable to sleep at night. She also noted clumsiness in her hands and the inability to use her arms well for any regular activities. Her right hand was much worse than the left. Jane was concerned she was not able to perform her job at the same pace she could previously. She was also worried about the loss of feeling in her hand.

Jane had probably performed her job for 20 years without complaint, and she wished to continue to do so. This woman, who worked to support herself, had a very strong work ethic. We brought Jane into our treatment program but in spite of conservative care in the way of splints, therapy, and lifestyle modification, she remained with severe symptoms.

Then a problem arose in the course of Jane's treatment; we were not able to obtain approval from her insurance carrier to move ahead with surgery. Before my eyes, I watched as her numbness became a more permanent fixture. The thenar muscles to her thumb were already dead.

Finally with the help of her attorney and an explanation to the judge, we were able to obtain approval to proceed with surgery for Jane. We not only released her ligament and freed the nerve at her carpal canal, but we also transferred one of her tendons to restore function of the thumb. Luckily, some sensation in her hand returned and showed markedly improved function. We were lucky to have been able to move forward in Jane's care. What this required was a thorough understanding on the part of Jane, the insurance carrier, and all others involved. Her ability to fight through the system, aggressively seeking this treatment before it was too late, saved this woman's hand.

It is important to remember pain, numbness, and tingling are simply your body's way of telling you something is wrong. These are warning signs and should not be ignored. On the other hand, nerves generally deteriorate over the course of months and years, and the fact these warning signs are there does not mean urgent, aggressive (operative) action must be taken. They are simply signs there is a problem to be addressed. The important thing is to find out just what is causing these symptoms and then take appropriate progressively aggressive actions to obtain relief from them.

Although numerous patients are given the diagnosis of carpal tunnel, many have much more significant problems with nerve involvement at other levels. Not all patients are candidates for surgery. In fact, some patients who have had surgery get no better or their condition worsens! Remember the following:

All that burns is not carpal tunnel.

"Lola" is a very talented artist who had complaints of nerve problems in her hands. She had been given multiple diagnoses including amyotrophic lateral sclerosis (Lou Gerhig's disease), ulnar neuropathy, and carpal tunnel syndrome. Unfortunately, in the process of making these diagnoses, her physicians never pursued any treatment. She developed severe wasting of the muscles in her hand, from both the ulnar and median nerves.

A stoic, uncomplaining woman, Lola continued to work as an artist and sculptor and created many outstanding works. But she had progressive problems and reached a point where she was unable to perform many of the manipulations required for her work. She had been able to compensate for the muscle wasting, but the numbness itself became a problem in that she was unable to use the hand because of the inability to feel what she was doing. Once her problem was correctly diagnosed, we performed surgery. This has been quite helpful in relieving some of her symptomatology, and she has had good early return of function in spite of her severe muscle atrophy.

What disturbed us more than anything else was her problem, although not painful, led her to become dysfunctional. Since her clinical picture was not "typical," she fell through the cracks of the system and very nearly lost all use of a wonderfully gifted hand. Although she had signs and symptoms of carpal tunnel and in fact a positive EMG for the same, Lola's main problem was her ulnar nerve at the elbow level. Had we operated on her carpal tunnel, this would not have given her good relief and would have been the wrong operation. Had she continued care under the diagnosis of carpal tunnel, I suspect today she would not be sculpting and would have a completely useless extremity. Fortunately, we were able to avert this but only by realizing her carpal tunnel was a secondary issue and not the primary problem.

Causation

The causes of carpal tunnel problems today are generally agreed upon. There is indeed a segment of the population predisposed to developing carpal tunnel and/or nerve problems. These are patients with underlying diseases and systemic diseases. Given the right situation and circumstances, they are more likely to develop problems with swelling and/or scarring of the nerves in the carpal canal. Medical conditions such as diabetes, hypothyroidism, hyperthyroidism, amyloidosis, and rheumatoid arthritis, to name a few, may result in increased inflammation or swelling of the structures in the carpal tunnel and/or altered circulation to the nerve and can cause symptoms consistent with a carpal tunnel–type problem.

Pregnancy and even menstruation during which there is significant fluid shifting may result in symptoms of carpal tunnel problems. In fact, it is very common during pregnancy for women to experience symptoms of carpal tunnel. These are almost invariably resolved once the child is delivered and the inflammation is gone. Traumatic issues that alter the biomechanics of the carpal canal such as broken or dislocated bones at the wrist level can result in decreased space in the carpal canal and production of symptoms in patients.

Simply having the above diseases or problems, however, does not in itself mean a patient will develop carpal tunnel. Although some of these issues may predispose a patient to having carpal tunnel problems there are many patients who have these diseases and problems and never develop carpal tunnel symptomatology or require treatment. It has been my experience patients develop nerve problems based on predictable insults or injuries to the nerves and tendon structures about the wrist and carpal tunnel area. Even if people with the above issues develop difficulties with less traumatic exposure, there is usually a causative factor for the development of these problems.

A patient who comes to mind is "William." A former Philadelphia fireman, he was cleaning leaves out of his gutters and fell off a ladder landing mostly on his right hand and wrist. His doctor sent him for X-rays, which reportedly showed no evidence of any broken bones or injury. Basically, he was told he just had a sprained wrist. However, he continued to be symptomatic with respect to severe pain and numbness in the hand.

I saw him in my office about three weeks after the incident. His complaints at that time were severe pain, discomfort, and swelling as well as numbness and tingling in his hand in the median nerve distribution. He also reported he could not move his fingers very well. He was in such pain, he would not let me touch him.

After meeting this gentleman, I was impressed by his significant pain issue. I had some concerns this might be an overreactive patient who was simply one of those "macho" types. He was a large man who appeared to have very little tolerance for pain. Upon examination, he indeed showed what appeared to be an injury to the wrist although his X-rays were reported as being normal.

We took additional X-rays that day and discovered he had dislocated his lunate bone (one of the eight bones in the wrist) into his carpal tunnel proper. This bone was so out of place it actually was sitting on the median nerve and causing direct compression and pressure. He had a volar lunate dorsal perilunate dislocation of the wrist. His original injury caused a tearing of his wrist ligaments. The early x-rays when reviewed showed some subtle change suggesting ligament damage. Over the next few days, the lunate completely dislocated, causing his symptoms.

We subsequently took him to surgery and after an extensive procedure relocated his lunate to its normal position and freed his median nerve in the carpal canal. He got excellent relief from his pain and discomfort, and we became good friends over the course of time.

A caveat to this story is at his six-month postoperative check-up appointment, which happened to fall on April 1, I met him in the exam room. He was sitting in the identical painful body posture I saw when he had first come to me and had his wrist wrapped in a splint. We had discussed over the course of the treatment the tendency for the lunate to dislocate recurrently in certain patients. This occurs when the ligaments do not heal rigidly enough. My color must have been ashen enough for him not to continue the joke and he looked up and said, "April fool." It seems he and my therapy staff decided to have some fun with me. He felt it only fair I join in a little bit of his suffering. (Although I was tempted to redislocate his wrist just on principle, I was able to control my urge and we all had a good laugh.)

Most individuals have an identifiable cause for median nerve problems. Motor vehicle accidents that result in a jamming of the hands on the wheel or patients who work with their hands on an aggressive basis such as using jackhammers or air or pneumatic tools are indeed predisposed and predictably will develop median nerve problems if using their hands long enough and aggressively enough. Patients who perform heavy labor activities such as rail workers or heavy laborers who use shovels, mallets, or hammers all day produce direct continued micro traumas or macro traumas to the nerves. They predictably will develop median nerve problems over the course of time. Those who regularly perform keyboard activities with repetitive fingering as well as repetitive wrist flexion/extension motion are also predisposed. Checkers who perform scanning and heavy lifting on a regular basis and others who use their hands, wrists, and arms repetitively with regular reaching, pulling, pushing, and flexion/ extension activities, such as in manufacturing lines, repeatedly traumatize the nerves resulting in inflammation and swelling. The actual number of motions is not as important as the continued motion with regular stresses being applied to the nerves.

"Tim" worked for the railroad for many years performing activities with his hands and arms, such as applying brakes which required turning a large wheel with all his strength. He also did a good deal of climbing and hanging onto railroad cars as they traveled. He subjected his upper arms to regular stresses on a repeated basis for many years and developed a classic cumulative trauma problem with progressive numbness, tingling, pain, and disability. He reached a point where he had severe problems with numbness in his hands and was unable to pursue any regular activities. He became significantly disabled, unable to pursue his work or his home avocations of cooking or playing the piano.

We evaluated Tim and discovered he had severe carpal tunnel problems as well as evidence of nerve involvement up higher in his arms. Therapy, splints, and altered activity were not helpful. Surgery, however, was successful in relieving his pain. He has continued to do well, but his arms are not normal. He has reached a point of livability but continues with limitations and cannot return to his previous occupation. If he had, he would no doubt have recurrent symptoms. He has taken an early retirement and is pursuing his piano and culinary activities.

I must state for the sake of completeness there are people who disagree with these concepts (of repeated traumas resulting in injury). It is popularly held in the medical community that regular insults to our nerves, joints, hearts, and minds are the factors that result in pathology. There are a few physicians who state carpal tunnel problems are just something people are born with and that life's regular traumas and daily activities do not result in these problems. This has not been my experience and is not consistent with logical thinking. The nature of science and scientific thinking is sequential; if there is a disease process and there is a reasonable causative factor, unless there is some other reason a person should develop problems, the cause-and-effect relationship should be considered the primary etiology.

Another issue that should appear self-evident is when we take patients out of the environment causing their symptoms, such as repetitive hand, wrist, and arm activities, and we do this prior to their developing significant scarring, they generally reverse the situation and do not require surgery. Certainly there is no 100-percent rule here but when evaluating the facts and overall conditions of our lives, we are usually able to identify the stressors that result in many of our symptoms, be they heart disease, ulcers, or carpal tunnel problems. It is simply a matter of honestly looking at each patient and his or her environment and determining how and why the cause and effect relationship exists.

A patient who comes to mind is "Jennie." She loved her job at a large investment company and spent many years performing phone and keyboard activities. Unfortunately, there was a merger in her company and she was transferred to the other company but performed the same activities. The only difference in the two jobs was the nonergonomic setup of her new work station and the amount of keying she performed. With the increased keying and her computer being set off to the side rather than directly in front of her causing a change in the position of her head and arm posturing, she had a rapid and progressive onset of symptoms. Jennie developed numbness and tingling in her hands and arms over the course of six weeks. There was no doubt a direct cause-and-effect relationship. When we modified her environment to its previous status, she became asymptomatic.

Unfortunately, every case is not as easy to recognize. All patients and employees are not as acutely aware of their own offending environmental factors, and their physicians are often not lucky enough to evaluate these cases early enough. When left to progress on the basis of continued inflammation and ultimate scarring, many patients require more intensive treatment than simply changing the position of the computer and work environment.

What Are Nerves Anyway?

CHAPTER 5

"I merely stir, press, feel with my fingers
and am happy; to touch my person
to someone else's is about as much
as I can stand."

—Walt Whitman

You may remember back in high school biology class when the teacher drew an axon and dendrite of a nerve similar to the one pictured in the figure. Your teacher told you this was a nerve; it was what made your entire body work. You learned these nerves are located throughout your body in your brain, spinal cord, arms, hands, and legs. They made your body act and react and were responsible for achieving every sort of physical and mental state from agony to ecstasy.

What your teacher may have failed to tell you is just how simple this system actually is. I spent the first year of medical school poring over physiology books trying to understand just how these little structures, which looked like amoebas, made things work. What I have come to understand is nerves function very much like electrical circuits. They simply conduct microcurrents of electricity from point A to point B.

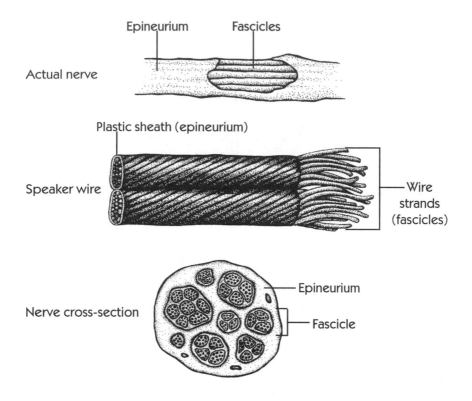

Nerves when viewed under a microscope look very much like speaker wire. The bottom drawing is a cross section through a nerve.

I find it helpful to use the analogy of electrical speaker wire to understand what nerves look like outside of our brain and spinal cord. The thin gold or silver strands of fine wire are analogous to the many fibers (fascicles) within the nerve sheath. The plastic coating on the outside of the speaker wire corresponds to the nerve sheath or epineurium.

Nerves actually look very much like this when viewed under a microscope. Although it would not be practical to wire a stereo system with our nerves, in essence the function is similar. These axon dendrite connections work in a similar manner to electrical wires. They conduct very low levels of electricity from our brain and spinal cord out to our fingertips and/or toes and then back again. The impulses come from the axon (cell body) and are transmitted through the dendrites.

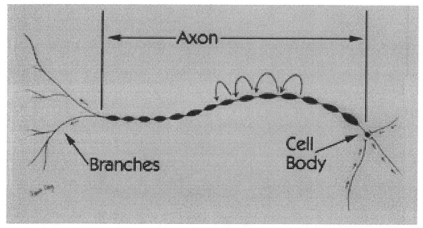

A peripheral nerve showing conduction of electrical impulses.

Nerve conduction involves a change in polarization which is a shift of positive and negative ions across a thin membrane. This shift is dependent on blood circulation and other related physiologic factors. Suffice it to say when this local shift cannot occur easily, the overall ability of that nerve to conduct electricity is compromised. This results in a slowing of the speed of conduction. When there is a delay in this speed of impulse conduction, which is predictable, the brain interprets this as abnormal and symptoms occur.

The key factor we need to understand is alterations in this capacity to conduct electricity are the basis of nerve problems. This alteration can be in the ability to conduct impulses *away* from the brain, resulting in disability in motor function, such as clumsiness, tremors, or weakness. Conversely, inability to conduct electricity in the opposite direction, i.e. from the fingers back to the spinal cord and brain causes a different scenario. When this reverse conduction becomes a problem, we experience numbness, tingling, altered sensation, and/or pain.

51

"Tina" found this out the hard way. She was working at a manufacturing plant and turned to place something on a table behind her. She caught her wrist on the sharp edge of an object and sustained a laceration to the small finger side of her wrist. She was seen in the emergency room and subsequently by a surgeon. She was taken to the operating room and an attempted repair of her nerve was done. The ulnar nerve itself was cut in half and she immediately lost sensation to her small finger and fourth digit. She also lost the fine motor control in the hand, which is supplied by the ulnar nerve, and the ability to move her fingers well.

Tina came to us and we performed nerve studies. These indicated she was getting no conduction across her nerve repair. Tina remained with severe pain and poor function in her hand. Our options were to allow her to continue to suffer and watch the hand deteriorate or to operate. Together we decided to go ahead with surgery. A new segment of nerve (graft) was placed to bridge the gap in her damaged nerve.

What is startling about these injuries is how rapidly function is lost; even more sobering is the devastation the patient experiences at the loss of use of a limb. This young woman was not only confronting pain but a dynamic shift in her life and future potential. Not only did she lose feeling but also lost the ability to perform fine motor functions with the hand. Using a fork, picking up change, even doing her hair became life challenges.

Following the surgery, she has had early progressive return of motor function and return of sensation but mostly a decrease in her pain. Her will to get better and her burning desire to heal have been inspirational.

Keep in mind the fact that anything that interferes with the normal operation of a nerve can produce pathology (symptoms). That is, if a nerve normally allows us feeling, power grip, and coordinated function (such as playing the piano), these functions could easily be lost if the nerve is functioning abnormally. The reason people have so many different types of symptoms when they have nerve problems is the symptoms produced depend upon which of the many nerve fibers are involved. For example, let's say we have an injury where the gold wire is cut. If the gold wire represents the sensory fibers leading from the thumb and silver to the rest of the hand, what will occur? This person will lose feeling to the thumb but there will be no effect on the rest of the hand. If we multiply this scenario by thousands of different fascicles (wires), then we see how confusing a particular patient's problem can appear to both patient and physician. On the other hand, if we as physicians (and patients) can simply look to identify which nerves are involved with the scarring or compression, the symptoms which we may consider at first to be inexplicable or bizarre become quite easily understood and logical.

"Gene" directed traffic with a construction crew. He had his back to oncoming traffic and was holding a stop/go sign to control traffic flow when a woman lost control of her car and ran directly into him. She knocked him up onto the hood and into her windshield. He was dazed and slid down off the front hood and ended up sitting with his back to the front bumper of her car. A second impact followed, and he was knocked off the road into a ditch.

Gene was helivac'd to an emergency trauma center. He sustained a number of injuries including unrelenting pain, numbness, and tingling in his hand, especially in his fourth and fifth fingers. He was told that nothing more could be done for him and he should just wait for his symptoms to go away. They did not; in fact, they got worse!

He had general evaluations and was told he did not have a carpal tunnel problem. This was self-evident to both Gene and me in that his pain and discomfort were at his elbow and his numbness was in his fourth and fifth digits, which are not the distribution of the carpal tunnel median nerve. We performed new EMG studies and looked at his ulnar nerve at the elbow. Gene had significant involvement here and a severely positive study indicating serious damage to the nerve.

We subsequently took Gene to surgery and he got excellent relief from his symptoms in the arm, and although he is not quite finished treatment, he is wonderfully improved with respect to his symptomatology. Here is a simple case of listening to the patient and hearing where the problem was. Once we heard his complaints were not carpal-tunnel related, we were easily able to identify the site of his nerve entrapment and give him relief. Thank goodness Gene had the fortitude to keep talking until someone heard what *he* had to say.

To further understand what can go wrong with nerves, we need to look again at basic nerve structure. The system begins in the brain which sends out an impulse. This comes out through the nerve roots from the spinal cord. Impulses of electricity are then transmitted along these nerves out to the end point receptors. These receptors can either be a muscle, which makes something move such as our fingers or arms, or an endpoint on the skin, which may control sweating or wrinkling. Nerves also go to the blood vessels and help control the amount of blood flow and circulation to the hand and arm.

Other nerve fibers send impulses from the distal hand and arm, such as the fingertips, back to the spinal cord and then up to the brain. These allow us to feel and sense our environment such as when we're being stuck with a needle or touch the hot burner of a stove. Luckily, when these nerves function normally, they can also bring us sensations of great joy, such as touching the face of a loved one. When these nerves function abnormally, the result can be an unbridled continuous release of sensory impulses to the brain, resulting in a pain syndrome.

When nerves become pathologically involved or a patient begins to have "nerve symptoms," it is because this ability of the nerve to conduct electricity from point A to point B has been compromised in some way. This compromise can occur anywhere along the path of the nerve from the spinal cord right down to the fingertips. This nerve impairment can result from local pressure or scarring.

When there is constriction or pressure on the nerve in one area only, local symptoms will occur, depending upon which nerve is involved. For instance, if a patient has a carpal tunnel problem, he or she may complain of pain as well as numbness or tingling of the hand in the median nerve distribution, which involves a thumb, index, long, and thumb side of the ring finger. When a nerve is so compromised, the associated symptoms will occur. We must remember, though, this nerve starts out in the neck; therefore, the symptoms may travel up into the arm and neck as well.

Nerves can be compromised in other ways. The epineurial sheath—discussed previously—can again be thought of as that plastic coating around the speaker wire. If this is frayed or defective and the wire is "wet" (scarred), then some of those fibers may be short-circuited. When this occurs, we may get static in our speakers or, in the case of nerves, altered function. This can reproduce different symptoms according to how significant the defect is and how the nerve is stimulated. Symptoms may be intermittent or constant and will vary in intensity. On a dry "good day," when there is no stress to the circuit, the nerve (wires) function fine. When it rains (a bad day), we will have a problem. This occurs in a like manner with nerves.

On a good day when nerves are not overstressed and overtaxed, they may function fine. On "bad" days, if there is a defect, they may act up significantly. Scar tissue about nerves does not allow them to move or glide well in their tissue beds. This scar can compromise the nerves' ability to function normally—either by yanking on the nerve when the hand or arm is moved or by essentially strangling the nerve and its blood supply.

Nerves can also be compromised at more than one level in the arm. When this occurs, it is often referred to as a double-crush syndrome or multi-level nerve involvement. Basically, the nerves are being pressed, pinched, or pulled (tractioned) at multiple sites. This is not uncommon and often results in a confusing clinical picture.

"Jennifer," a teacher, music therapist and a highly dynamic individual, presented to us as a patient who had significant problems with her left arm. Jennifer had spent many years working by playing guitar as well as piano. Music was her work and a big part of her life. Initially, her complaint was consistent with a carpal tunnel problem. The problem was numbness and tingling in her hand and pain and discomfort radiating up her arm.

She developed progressive symptoms and on further evaluation, it became apparent her problem was not simply at the carpal tunnel. She had scarring about her median nerve not only at the wrist and hand level but also in her forearm between the elbow and wrist. It was evident she had involvement at the brachial plexus level between the neck and shoulder as well. When we began Jennifer's treatment, it became apparent early on she had substantial involvement at all these levels with severe scarring about these nerves. When she placed her arms in different positions and postures (stressing the nerves), this resulted in reproduction of her numbness, tingling, and pain.

This is a highly motivated individual who presented a significantly confusing clinical picture. Once we were able to sort things out, it became apparent she had substantial nerve involvement at many levels. Due to the severity of her pain, it was necessary to free all of these nerves to give her enough relief to move forward with her life. Jennifer has been through three surgeries freeing the nerves from her wrist and hand all the way to her thoracic outlet or brachial plexus level. She has had excellent relief from the surgeries and, in fact, has gone back to work.

Let's continue our example and compare a nerve to a garden hose. You are out in your yard on a bright, sunny day watering your garden. One of your neighbors comes along and starts a conversation with you. Inadvertently, she stands on the hose while you are watering. You may not notice any significant change in the flow through your hose and continue to water your garden while the conversation continues. The flow remains adequate because the amount of pressure on the hose (or nerve) is not too great at this point. This is similar to the person who has a low level nerve problem, who is essentially stable and not symptomatic.

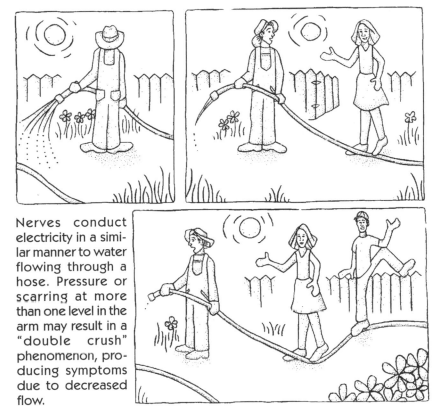

Nerves conduct electricity in a similar manner to water flowing through a hose. Pressure or scarring at more than one level in the arm may result in a "double crush" phenomenon, producing symptoms due to decreased flow.

Now, let us get back to our gardening. While carrying on this conversation with your neighbor, her husband hops over the fence and joins in the conversation. Unfortunately, he too stands on the hose, a few feet down the line. Suddenly, you interrupt your conversation when you realize there is not enough flow to water your plants. Your neighbor and husband have compromised the flow in the hose and constitute a double-crush–type problem. There is now pressure on your hose, or nerve, at two levels. The flow has been cut down to the point where this becomes noticeable or "symptomatic." Likewise, if the hose were pulled and stretched with force, it would narrow. The result of this yanking or twisting would be comparable to a traction type phenomenon with nerves resulting again in decreased flow and symptoms.

Applying this example to the nerves of the upper extremities, we usually see double-crush involvement at a level up by the neck and also down by the wrist or hand. When this occurs, we have a dangerous situation. The overall flow and speed of electrical conduction have been slowed to the point which the brain interprets as a significant delay in impulse conduction. This manifests as numbness, pain, tingling, or weakness. These poor victims of multi-level nerve involvement are often labeled with incomplete diagnoses, or worse as "treatment failures" if they still have symptoms after carpal tunnel surgery.

Indeed this is the injustice suffered by many patients who have "simple" nerve problems or what is thought to be "just" carpal tunnel. They do not improve or get better. The "predictable" simple surgery never cures these patients and many are labeled as treatment failures. The problem is not with the patient or, at times, with the operation. It is simply only one level of compression has been relieved but that was not the most symptomatic point. It is unfortunate but often instead of looking further, we as physicians, send these patients away to the next program rather than trying harder to understand the real problem.

When you understand how nerves function, you will realize someone who continues to have pain even though the medical community has done "everything" is not at the end. Doctors are not always right, and at times, just don't understand. Doctors are people and can only take a patient as far as their individual understanding will allow. I always tell my patients not to let a doctor stifle their innate abilities to heal. If one physician can't help bring out their inner capabilities, there is almost always another who can. Remember to try and fail is admirable but to not even try is unforgivable. Your doctor must help you try.

I had an interesting experience a number of years ago while giving a lecture to a group of doctors on our technique for carpal tunnel surgery. After my presentation, I was asked a question by one of the attending orthopedic surgeons. He asked me why I was making such a big deal over new techniques for carpal tunnel surgery. He told me he had performed this operation the same way for many years and none of his patients had ever had a problem.

I asked him how he was able to obtain such wonderful results. He told me he had never had a patient come back and tell him they had recurrent problems or any residual symptoms after surgery. He told me he sent them back to work one week post-operatively, and there was no need for him to see them after that. Another doctor got up from the audience and told him, "Of course they don't come back; they went somewhere else!" Obviously, this doctor had no understanding of nerve problems. Further, he did not educate his patients as to the possibility of long-term problems or recurrence of scarring—substantial issues in nerve disease.

The illustration indicates how these nerves start at the cervical spine. They leave as nerve roots and form a complex network called the brachial plexus. Every nerve that goes into the hand and arm travels through it. The three major nerves in the arm—the median, radial, and ulnar—arise from the brachial plexus. They separate into individual nerves at about the shoulder level and then go down the arm to the hand and wrist. The median nerve gives us sensation or feeling to the thumb,

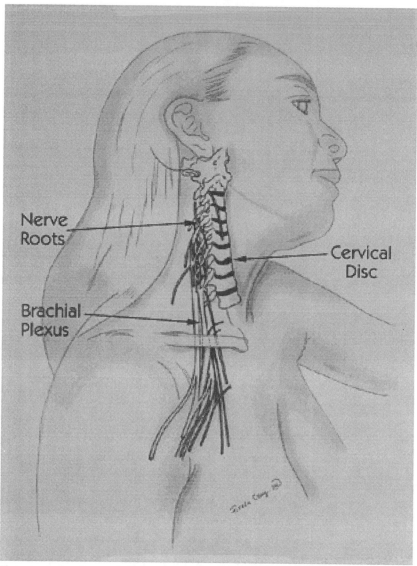

The cervical spine and discs are seen in their normal anatomic alignment. The nerve roots exit the spine and form the nerves of the brachial plexus. These travel through the thoracic outlet to form the major nerves of the arm.

the index and long fingers, and radial half (or thumb side) of the fourth or ring finger. The median nerve also supplies motor function to those muscles that help us make a fist and the ab-ductor pollicis brevis muscle that allows us to oppose the thumb.

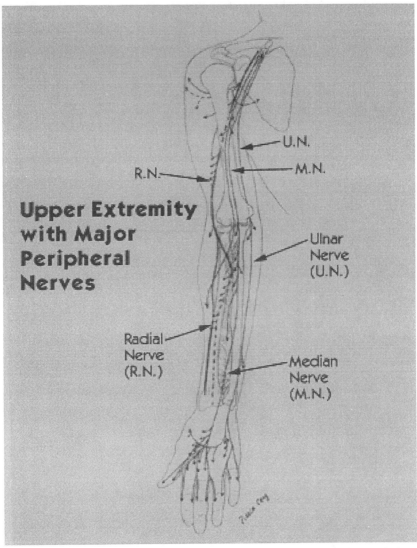

U.N.

M.N.

R.N.

Upper Extremity with Major Peripheral Nerves

Ulnar
Nerve
(U.N.)

Radial
Nerve
(R.N.)

Median
Nerve
(M.N.)

The nerves of the upper extremity begin as the thoracic outlet and then travel as long cables from the neck to the fingertips. The three nerves inner-vating the hand: the median, radial and ulnar are seen here in their entirety. Pathology at any level can produce symptoms throughout the arm.

61

The ulnar nerve travels down the arm behind the elbow and into the hand giving us sensation to the small and little finger side of the ring finger. This controls fine motor function in the hand and dexterity.

The radial nerve allows us to bring our fingers out straight and our wrists back. This runs down the arm on the outside of the elbow. This controls the extensor muscles of the forearm and also gives us sensation on the back of the hand.

As you can see, the nerves in the arm make up a very well-designed mechanism. When functioning well, this is a wonderfully coordinated mechanism that orchestrates activities from eating and hunting to playing a piano concerto. Through these nerves and our hands, we can experience all the wonderful things in the world. Conversely, when they are not functioning well, they can make our lives miserable.

Nerves may also be compromised at the level of the neck by occurrences such as disc herniations. These decrease the ability of the nerve to conduct electricity by direct pressure. Discs are cushions between the vertebrae (bones) of the neck and spinal column. These discs have soft material inside called the nucleus pulposus. There is a harder, outer portion called the annulus fibrosis. If a patient has a severe whiplash-type injury or a significant crunching or crush injury to the head and neck, this inner portion, the nucleus pulposus, may be pushed out to the side, pressing on the nerve at the neck nerve root. It is important to remember, however, patients with nerve problems at the neck level do not necessarily have "herniated discs." It is even more vital to be aware a negative magnetic resonance imaging (MRI) scan showing no disc involvement does not tell the whole story.

In many cases, nerves can be injured at the level of the thoracic outlet. Remember the brachial plexus contains all the nerves that go into the arm. This connects the nerve root at the neck to the upper arm and the plexus spans the gap between the neck and shoulder. The tunnel or outlet through which the nerves of the brachial plexus travel is called the thoracic outlet. Compromise at this level can reproduce almost any symptom or sensation normally produced by these nerves. The clinical picture may be quite confounding and often the diagnosis is difficult to make. Thoracic Outlet Syndrome can be a tremendously disabling and difficult problem to treat. (A later chapter is devoted to brachial plexus problems and the details of treatment.)

"Steve" is a man who worked his life in construction. Although at one point he had a supervisory position, he had to change jobs and began working manual labor again using a jackhammer and pneumatic air tools. Due to repeated exposure to the vibratory tools, his hands, wrists, shoulders, and neck were traumatized. Because he developed severe progressive painful problems with numbness in his arms, he became unable to perform this work. He had severe nerve damage involving the median nerve at the wrist, ulnar nerve at the elbow, and scarring about the nerves at his brachial plexus. Although MRI scans had been done to rule out a disc problem in his neck, his pain was not coming from a cervical spine injury but rather from the scarring of the nerves about his brachial plexus. The cumulative traumas induced by the weight of the jackhammer and the repeated yanking and vibratory injury resulted in severe scarring of the nerves about his brachial plexus.

It was only through understanding the history of the type of insults he sustained and a thorough evaluation as well as electrical studies that we were able to ascertain this gentleman not only was sane but indeed had severe pain due to underlying physiologic nerve disease and scarring. Taking Steve out of this environment has at least been partially helpful in giving him some relief.

Distally or in the far end of the arm, each of the nerves described previously—the median, radial, and ulnar—has its own compression syndromes and problems. Each of these is generally a localized compression and can produce symptoms unique to that individual nerve.

The medical community has not been aggressive enough in educating the public about nerve disease. In fact, there is controversy among members of the medical community as to the exact pathophysiology of many of the problems discussed here. Today, because of a number of factors, multi-level nerve problems are much more commonly diagnosed. Occupations requiring repetitive motions using high speed technology, such as scanners in grocery stores, computers, and high-speed machines in manufacturing plants have contributed to the stresses on nerves, tendons, and joints.

With high-powered engines, younger drivers, and increased speed limits, car accidents now occur at increasingly higher speeds. Seat belts are very helpful and absolutely do save lives! Unfortunately, they also change the way the forces are transmitted through our bodies tractioning both the neck and the brachial plexus. This results in significant and severe yanking or tractioning injuries. Thus increased mechanization in our society has indeed created new ways to compromise nerves due to injury and repetitive traumas.

More than likely we all know someone who has had carpal tunnel or some other nerve surgery and has "failed at medical treatment." The blame is placed *on the patient* and not our lack of medical knowledge and capabilities. The fact is, many of these patients have significant nerve disease that has gone undiagnosed. These are patients with real pain and physiologic disease. The fact the medical community often cannot isolate the specifics of the nerve compression problem relegates these patients to being labeled as "chronic pain patients" rather than patients with "true" disease.

Forty-year-old "Tammy" came to me in a severely depressed state. Her job at an automobile manufacturer required repetitive activities with her upper extremities. She had progressive problems with neurologic compromise resulting in an inability to use her hands and arms. By that time her pain and nerve symptoms progressed to the point where she had basically become afunctional and demoralized due to her inability to work. To make matters even worse, her father passed away. She became deeply depressed.

With the help of conservative care and treatment with therapy and biofeedback training, Tammy has made a wonderful recovery. She pulled herself up and went back to school and pursued training for a completely new career. A mature woman who had never before attended college, she achieved a 3.8 grade average. Although her pain and symptomatology still do exist, they are at a much lower level. She has been able to modify her life to live within her limitations. We gave her little more than a diagnosis, therapy, and an understanding of her disease, but with encouragement and knowledge she began to control her nerve problems and develop more faith in herself. We also assured her the symptoms and problems she had were real.

Tammy's situation is an example of a serious problem in our community today. If you are a nerve pain sufferer, then you need to know the majority of people who have nerve pain have it for physiologic and not psychological reasons. That is not to say every patient with pain has a nerve compression problem, but it has been my experience most people who have pain have some physiologic basis for that pain. Once we can isolate the source of this pain and teach patients how to modify their lives and activities, it can usually be controlled if not eliminated. Sometimes it is necessary to surgically "free" these nerves to allow them to heal, but the key factor to remember here is nerves do heal and get better and pain does go away!

In summary, the basic function of the nervous system is relatively simple, and unless the nerve is cut, there should be a way to make it function properly. All a nerve needs to function properly is to conduct electricity from point A to point B. When pain exists due to malfunction of nerves, the key is to find out where the conduction block or delay is and simply allow normal function to return. It is sometimes a lengthy and painstaking process, but in most cases it is achievable.

Physicians have been advised to "heal thyself." Perhaps, the more correct advice here would be for the patient in pain: "If your physician cannot even heal himself, show him or her how to heal you!"

The Diagnosis
of Nerve Problems

CHAPTER 6

Doctors are trained basically as scientists. Ideally, diagnoses should be arrived at through a reproducible method based on scientific thinking and protocols. Nerves, however, do not lend themselves easily to this concept. Patients often present with confounding clinical pictures, frustrating not only themselves but their treating physicians as well. This contributes to the great amount of controversy in diagnosis and treatment programs for nerve problems.

As any first-year medical student will tell you, the basis of a good diagnosis and treatment plan depends on a good history. It is imperative when evaluating any patient to obtain a thorough understanding of the patient's history, including a look at that person's life activities. A thorough history of previous insults and injuries over the years should also be taken. A previous history of a bad wrist fracture or direct trauma to the carpal tunnel, for example, can produce symptoms consistent with a median nerve or carpal tunnel problem. This can be secondary to direct pressure, scarring, or alteration of the biomechanics of the carpal tunnel.

This reminds me of a story I heard early in my career that emphasizes the importance of knowing a patient's history. A study was conducted to evaluate the incidence of cervical cancer in various populations. It was noted there was a high correlation between the development of cancer of the cervix and sexual promiscuity. Multiple semen exposures resulted in a much higher risk of cervical cancer in these individuals. However, to make this matter confusing, the highest incidence of cervical cancer in an isolated population was found in a convent. Obviously, this threw a monkey wrench into the theoretical correlation between sex and the cancer. This is where taking a more thorough history became important.

It seems this convent was actually a home for wayward women and most of the women at this convent had previously had colorful lives. They had come to the convent to repent their ways. What appeared to be a contradiction of the original hypothesis was actually confirmation. This was an isolated group of high-risk individuals whose previous sexual promiscuity was a contributing and causative factor in their disease processes. Without this piece of information in the history, it would be difficult if not impossible to isolate this group as high risk.

Motor vehicle accidents such as whiplash injuries or flexion/extension injuries can also result in nerve involvement at the neck or thoracic outlet level between the neck and shoulder. This results from a tractioning or yanking of the nerves from their normal beds. If the resultant inflammation causes scarring about the nerves, patients may remain with symptoms or limitations in motion which set up the possibility of injury from lesser stresses in the future.

"Abe" is a highly successful businessman and also an airplane pilot. He came to me with the diagnosis of a carpal tunnel problem. We talked extensively and he told me his major problems were when he held his neck in certain postures. Looking up or in certain directions caused his arm to go numb. He gave a classic description of a cervical spine involvement and on further evaluation and investigation, it was noted he had significant disc disease at the neck level. If he drives long distances and does not rest and stretch, his hands go numb. He has made substantial lifestyle modifications. His problem of severe pain and discomfort is now not only livable but he has made himself quite functional.

He has found by changing the position of the seats in his car as well as his airplane (which actually is a more comfortable seat for him), he is able to perform all activities without reproducing his numbness. If his original presumed diagnosis of carpal tunnel had been pursued and he had carpal tunnel surgery, he would at best have had partial relief. Without full evaluation and treatment of his neck problem, treatment would most likely have led only to frustration.

The importance of history cannot be overemphasized. All too often, we as doctors don't understand our patients prior to undertaking treatment with them. What seems a small or incidental piece of information can often be the difference between successful treatment and failure or worse.

I remember a patient from years ago who had been on insulin and complained of multiple episodes of insulin shock, a dangerous condition if left unchecked. She unquestioningly followed her doctor's advice to the letter of the law, and when instructed to take her insulin every morning, she did so. However, there was one piece of critical information left out of her history: She worked nights. She ate her meals during the course of the night (her daytime) and in the morning would come home and go to sleep. Unfortunately, this meant she was taking her insulin at exactly the wrong time. It was not until this part of her history was discovered her insulin dosages were adjusted appropriately and she stopped having these episodes.

Further historic issues to be examined are a history of juvenile-onset diabetes, thyroid disease, pregnancy, or other systemic problems that can cause either alteration of the circulation to the nerves proper or increased swelling at the level of the carpal tunnel. The history should be detailed as to any other injuries, problems, or the type of symptoms the patient exhibits. A patient who has problems with overhead activities, head positioning, or posturing may have a neck, upper arm, or brachial plexus problem rather than solely a carpal tunnel problem. Conversely, a patient who has problems with wrist and hand positioning and increased problems with activities such as typing, keying, gripping, or the like, likely has a local problem at the wrist or hand level.

After taking a complete history, a physical examination should be performed. This examination would include a number of tests to determine where the major point of scarring or entrapment of the nerve may be. It is important to point out an examination for an upper extremity nerve problem should be from head to fingertips. Today the pressures of managed care impose time limitations on physicians. For example, patients who complain of numbness in the hand are often simply evaluated at that level only. An examination is done at the hand and wrist and a "partial" diagnosis of a problem at the carpal tunnel may be made. I've seen this unfortunate mistake many times. The patient is never examined above the elbow until well after two or even three surgeries have failed. It is only at that time the physicians may begin to look proximally at the neck or thoracic outlet level for other involvements.

"Carl" is a young man who worked as an electroplater, which consisted of a great deal of reaching activity with his upper arms pulling, pushing, and lifting heavy plates out and away from him. This caused a significant amount of stress on his upper neck and brachial plexus. He developed progressive problems with pain and discomfort in his neck and shoulder and into his arm. He was awakened with this pain and subsequently underwent surgery by a prominent neurosurgeon for a disc problem in his neck. Carl got some relief with the surgery but it was incomplete. His significant arm and neck pain continued, and the surgeon told him his pain was psychological in origin. The doctor did not want to hear his patient still had pain after "successful disc surgery."

We evaluated Carl and believed his problem was not at his neck but at his lower arm and brachial plexus. He subsequently underwent median nerve surgery at the wrist and thoracic outlet surgery. Carl got very good relief from his pain and discomfort. Unfortunately, although he was doing very well post-operatively, due to substantial stress in his home life, his recovery faltered.

Clearly, if we hadn't examined Carl's whole life, we would not have been able to evaluate his medical problems. Here is a person who had not only disease at his neck level but also outside the neck at the brachial plexus. He had successful surgery and continues to be symptomatic. The major issue he faces at this point is stabilizing his home situation. Without knowledge of this and a thorough understanding of the same, it would be impossible to help him by just treating his body. His current pain is inextricably intertwined with his psyche. Carl has pain on both a physical and an emotional level. Although his physical pain has been treated and is improved, Carl will only heal completely when he is mentally prepared to do so.

Physical Examination

A detailed examination includes an evaluation for range of motion of hands, wrists, elbows, shoulders, and neck for rotation and side bending. It is important to determine if there is a limitation of motion and if there is pain at the extremes of motion. These are helpful in evaluating for joint problems as well as nerve involvement. Many patients avoid motion because it is painful. Some motions, such as raising the shoulder, actually pull on the nerves of the brachial plexus and increase symptoms.

The following are a few of the tests used to evaluate patients with nerve problems and to indicate at which level problems are present.

Tinel's Testing

The Tinel sign is a test that evaluates patients for inflammation, swelling, or irritability of a nerve. Most of the nerves of the body can be palpated or felt because they are fairly superficial beneath the skin. This can be used to our advantage in diagnostic testing by either tapping lightly or pressing on these nerves. A Tinel's sign should be elicited by light and gentle tapping. Those who attempt to do this with a reflex hammer or aggressive methods are risking overresponse and diffuse pain, which are not helpful in evaluating nerve symptoms.

A Tinel's sign is elicited by lightly tapping over a nerve and simply asking the patient, "What do you feel?" If the patient relates radiation of numbness, tingling, burning, or nerve sensations, which are termed dysesthesias, and this is in an appropriate distribution for that nerve, this would be considered a positive test. For instance, tapping at the median nerve at the wrist level may elicit numbness, tingling, or sensation in the distribution of that nerve to the thumb, index, long, and possibly thumb side of the ring finger. One or any of these fingers involved may constitute a positive response. Some patients actually relate radiation of pain proximally up into the arm, which indicates there may be nerve involvement proximally at the forearm or brachial plexus level.

This same test can be performed at the ulnar nerve at the wrist and the ulnar nerve at the elbow, which is the "funny bone" nerve. The radial nerve at the wrist may also be irritable at the thumb side, indicative of pathology here as well.

Tinel signs can be elicited at the thoracic outlet or brachial plexus level. These would be in the supraclavicular (above the collarbone) or infraclavicular (below the collarbone) areas as described previously. They are evaluated by pressing lightly with the examiner's thumbs. If the patient relates radiation of the nerve symptoms into the arm, this may indicate scarring or inflammation about the nerves of the brachial plexus.

Testing by compression or distraction of the neck may indicate nerve root or disc problems.

Phalen's Test

The Phalen's test is performed by holding the patient's wrist in a flexed or bent down position for 60 seconds, or bent up in a reversed Phalen's test in what I call the prayer position for 60 seconds. Again, the patient should be asked, "What do you feel?" This may test for median and/or ulnar nerve symptoms at the wrist level in that this puts increased pressure on the median and ulnar nerve at the wrist. Positive response indicates pathology generally at the wrist and hand level or the carpal tunnel.

Elbow Flexion Test

The elbow flexion test is done by having the patient bend his elbows up completely and holding this position for 60 seconds. This may elicit symptoms in the ulnar nerve distribution indicating a problem possibly with the ulnar nerve at the elbow.

Compression Test

A compression test can be performed by either having the examiner press and hold pressure on the median nerve or ulnar nerve at the wrist or forearm, or by using a blood pressure cuff on the forearm. This may reproduce numbness and tingling usually testing the median or ulnar nerve. This is another test, if performed appropriately, that can be helpful in localizing nerve pathology. Again the test should be performed for a full 60 seconds.

Tension Tests for Brachial Plexus Problems

There are a number of tests used to determine pathology or scarring about the nerves of the brachial plexus. The most commonly used tests are the Wright's, Hunter's, EAST (elevated arm stress test), and Roos tests. These are all performed by having the patient assume various positions with arms raised above the head or down below and to the sides. The examiner may ask the patient to turn his or her head to one side or another to help further elicit symptomatology. Different postures at the wrists and elbows may be asked for as well to reproduce traction on different trunks of the brachial plexus. It is important for the patient to hold this position for at least 60 seconds. These tests are very helpful in evaluating nerve scarring and/or compression problems of the nerves at the brachial plexus.

Adson's Test

The Adson's test is misunderstood today. This is done by having the patient extend the arms out and either up and away from the body or down and away as the examiner checks the patient's pulse when the patient turns his or her head to one side or another and takes a deep breath. A decrease or change in pulse can be helpful in determining if there is a vascular (circulation) component to the brachial plexus problem. It is important to remember only about 3 percent of brachial plexus problems are vascular. Maintenance of a pulse does not rule out a thoracic outlet problem. The subclavian artery supplies most of the circulation to the arm and shares the same "tunnel" as the nerves in the thoracic outlet. If there is a vascular component to the pathology, it usually means there is severe compression of both blood vessels and nerves.

These are the major tests used to determine if nerve pathology is present. Many patients have difficulty in describing nerve symptoms; I have had descriptions of nerve symptoms varying from numbness, tingling, burning, "funny feelings," hot flashes, and shooters to "loss of circulation" or a cold sensation in the hand or fingers. All of these responses are appropriate. Sometimes the term dysesthesias, or altered sensations, is used rather than trying to pin this down to a specific burning or numbness and tingling issue. It is important to note if symptoms are produced and these are similar symptoms to those the patient experiences when they have complaints, these tests could and should be considered positive.

"Betty" came in with what she thought were simple carpal tunnel problems. She was correct about one arm, but there were significant nerve issues from her hand all the way up to her brachial plexus level on the other arm. She had excellent relief on the original side but surgery on the opposite hand did not help her upper arm and significant symptoms and problems continued. She has been through a prolonged course of therapy treatment as well as training in biofeedback and pain-management techniques.

Betty has reached a point where she believes her symptoms are definitely improved. She has made extensive lifestyle modifications to make her disease livable. She avoids all the positions and postures that irritate her arms. Betty has made understanding her disease a strength, and she uses this knowledge to modify her daily routines so she does not exacerbate her underlying problem. She is an excellent example of a patient who has gone on to lead a relatively normal life in spite of having significant, multi-level nerve disease.

It is important also to remember everyone with positive testing does not have severe pathology. The history, examination, and entire clinical picture must be correlated to determine whether there is simply nerve irritability or actual nerve pathology requiring aggressive treatment. The examination must be thorough and evaluate all the nerves at all levels so a complete picture can be put together.

Radiographs (X-rays)

Radiographs, or X-rays, are another useful tool in the diagnosis of nerve problems. X-rays are valuable in determining if there are major alterations in the contour of the carpal tunnel and also to rule in or out any bone spurs or ligament instability patterns at the wrist level. They are also quite helpful in determining whether there is a secondary component of involvement at the neck level with arthritis, narrowing of the disc space, or cervical ribs. Often bony abnormalities can help us in predicting other levels of nerve involvement.

The history, examination, and baseline X-rays should generally be enough to rule on a diagnosis of either carpal tunnel or another level of nerve involvement. The following tests should be used as confirmatory tests of the diagnosis and to help pin down a treatment plan.

Magnetic Resonance Imaging

MRI scanners have become quite helpful in diagnosing a number of different problems and maladies. Discs which are the spacers between the bones of the neck can be seen quite readily on MRI scans. Bulges or herniations pressing on nerve roots (where they leave the spinal cord) can often be detected. They can*not*, however, tell us how these nerves are functioning.

MRIs are helpful at times in ruling in or out ligament injuries at the wrist level. They can also tell us if there is tendinitis in the carpal canal. But an MRI read as positive for carpal tunnel syndrome should be taken with a grain of salt. Although we can at times see some changes in the shape of the carpal tunnel and the nerve in the carpal canal, the MRI itself has not yet been shown to be diagnostic of clinically significant carpal tunnel problems. That is, if you have only an MRI scan that says you have carpal tunnel syndrome, don't jump into surgery solely on the basis of a radiographic finding.

Electromyelography/Nerve Conduction Velocity

EMG/nerve conduction studies are tests performed to help validate suspected nerve problems. Recording electrodes and acupuncture-type needles are placed in the arm and neck areas and the nerve is pulsed with an electrical shock to see how well it conducts electricity. This determines the nerve's ability to conduct electricity from one point to another. If indeed there is slowing of this speed or velocity, there is generally a problem with the nerve such as compression or scarring of the nerve. The test may be uncomfortable but in the right hands can be a very valuable tool in evaluating complex nerve problems.

I often have patients indicate to me they know they are ready to have surgery because they are ready to risk a new EMG/NCV. A good friend of mine who is also a nurse often gives me a hard time when it comes to this. She had a number of surgeries on her arms.

When I ask her how she is feeling, she generally says, "Not bad enough to have a new EMG." This is often a good predictor of just how much discomfort a patient is having. The test is uncomfortable and patients who've already had one EMG/NCV usually relate willingness or unwillingness to have another based on the amount of discomfort they are suffering at that point in time.

If the EMG/NCV findings are consistent with the problem and help to confirm this, then indeed surgery *may* be indicated. EMG/NCVs may also be helpful in localizing where surgery should be performed. They can help determine whether the problem is at the level of the carpal tunnel, the elbow, or even higher up at the neck or brachial plexus level.

However, just because a patient has a positive EMG/NCV for a nerve problem does not mean he or she requires aggressive treatment. In fact, as you will see in later chapters, EMG/NCVs can go from positive (pathologic) to negative (normal) with judicious conservative treatment. Nerves have a wonderful innate capacity to heal themselves. It is well documented that a high percentage of the people in the general population past the age of 35 to 40 have positive EMG/NCV studies and no symptoms. These patients do not require surgery either.

A word of caution about EMG/NCV studies: These studies are highly variable and done by a number of different professionals. Physiatrists, neurologists, physical therapists, and others perform EMG/NCV studies. The study itself is a technical one and is only as good as the examiner. There are many nerve problems in the arms that are difficult to evaluate via electrical studies. A negative EMG/NCV that does not confirm or show the problem does not rule out the presence of a problem. At times, an EMG/NCV may be negative and indeed the problem may not exist. At other times, the EMG/NCV may be positive and yet clinically the patient has no symptoms. If a patient is symptomatic and the examiner is not able to document these symptoms on EMG/NCV, this simply means either there is not enough scarring about the nerve for the EMG/NCV to be positive at that time or possibly the examiner is not capable of studying the nerve specifically at that level. An EMG/NCV study is most helpful when the patient has clinical symptoms and the examination, history, and nerve conduction studies are all consistent.

"Dan," a 48-year-old, right-hand-dominant machinist, was working on a bar press. As he was pulling it down fairly hard, the bar jammed and did not complete its travel. He felt and heard a crack in his right wrist and had pain and discomfort in the wrist, up the arm, and into the neck. His arm actually went numb at the time of the incident and he had significant swelling and pain in the wrist and hand and was unable to use the arm after the incident. Dan was subsequently diagnosed as having a fracture in the wrist and also a nerve problem in his arm—labeled carpal tunnel—and tendinitis in his thumb. Carpal tunnel surgery was performed and his wrist was put into a cast. Dan continued to be quite symptomatic and had no relief at all with the surgery. The pain in his hand continued and radiated up his arm. He was losing strength in his arm and hand, and he continued having numbness and tingling in his thumb and third and fourth fingers in addition to a sharp pain on the palm side of the wrist. He was out of work for 13 weeks after the initial injury and another 6 weeks after his carpal tunnel surgery. He had been sent back to work using the hand minimally.

Dan subsequently came under our care. His rehabilitation nurse through his workmen's compensation carrier had appropriately diagnosed him as having a significant problem in his right arm. After talking with Dan and given her experience with patients having significant nerve problems, she realized he did not simply have a carpal tunnel problem. Dan entered our therapy program and underwent further surgery, ultimately requiring thoracic outlet surgery. Indeed, this is where his problem originated. He had sustained a significant tractioning or yanking injury to the nerves of his brachial plexus. He developed severe scarring and pressure on the nerves up at the level where they leave the spinal cord between the neck and shoulder proper. Although his symptoms were similar to those of other patients with carpal tunnel syndrome, there were some significant differences. Dan related pain and discomfort radiating all the way up his arm to his neck level and symptoms with motion of the entire arm. He also had an injury consistent with an upper arm problem.

Dan came to me with a story that made sense. His symptoms, complaints, and history of injury were all consistent with a significant nerve problem in his right arm. He told me what his problem was and ultimately how to fix it. It was in essence the relationship and communication between Dan and me that allowed us to ultimately get him relief and cure his problem. It took a joint effort on the part of Dan, his rehabilitation nurse, and our staff to come to a firm diagnosis and ultimately bring him good relief with the correct surgical treatment.

One caveat is Dan's arm is still not normal. Although he has gotten excellent relief from his pain and discomfort and has gone back to regular use of his arm, we have been careful to emphasize his is indeed not a normal arm. The key is he understands his disease and limitations and needs to protect this hand and arm in the long term. Dan understands if he does tax this or goes back to the type of activities he performed previously as a machinist, then he will no doubt have recurrent problems and require further treatment or there may be no treatment left that would give him any relief.

Dan had the wherewithal to continue to seek treatment in spite of "failed carpal tunnel surgery." He became a treatment success due to his persistent belief in himself and the persistent belief in him by others. He was finally able to understand his disease and his symptoms and help us put together a well thought out and agreeable treatment plan.

As stated earlier in this chapter, the cornerstone of making a diagnosis of nerve problems in the upper extremities is the history and examination. A complete history and exam done at the initial sitting are imperative in that over the course of time, problems can become more confusing and confounding. It is also important, no matter where you are in the course of your treatment, you find someone who is willing to sit down and take the time to perform a full and comprehensive evaluation from head and neck to fingertips. Unless this is done, many oversights occur and at times treatment will be rendered in a less than optimal manner. At times surgeries are done based on incomplete diagnoses and unrealistic expectations of both patient and surgeon. The additional studies talked about in this chapter including the MRI and EMG/NCV are simply confirmatory tests to help solidify clinical suspicions. No one test or diagnostic tool should be taken as definitive. Unless the whole picture makes sense, the treatment won't either!

The Conservative
Treatment of Nerve Pain

CHAPTER 7

*"I know of no more encouraging fact than
the unquestionable ability of man to elevate
his life by a conscious endeavor."*

–Henry David Thoreau

The obvious question you should ask yourself is why I, a surgeon, am writing a chapter on the conservative treatment of carpal tunnel and nerve problems. Indeed this is a question I have asked myself many times. Being a surgeon is one of the most challenging and rewarding professions one could hope to undertake. As a surgeon, I have the unique opportunity to fully evaluate and treat patients in many ways. I begin with a thorough history and physical examination. Through this, I am hopefully able to understand what my patients are feeling and through my examination become familiar with their tissues, scarring, and pathology. I can then prescribe a conservative treatment program in the way of therapy, lifestyle and behavior modification. This is called conservative treatment.

If my patient remains symptomatic, I can obtain further information through testing such as EMG and nerve conduction studies as well as X-rays and possibly even MRI scanning when appropriate. These give me a further understanding of the nature of my patients' injuries and insults. We have the opportunity at this point to either modify the conservative plan or to consider more aggressive interventions in the way of injections, splints, or stronger medication.

When all else fails, I have the most valued privilege of all. I can actually operate and look inside my patient's body to see whether my clinical impression, the diagnostic studies, and my patient's pathology are consistent and make sense. I have the outstanding opportunity to look at the nerves and hopefully remedy or lessen the disease present. I have the advantage of actually seeing, feeling, touching, holding, and moving these structures. I can view the scar tissue and observe how this effects the nerves. I am able to observe the effect of releasing ligaments and scar from about these structures.

When I write about nerve problems and pathology, I am not just relating research or animal studies. I am reporting the real thing; what we actually see inside the human body.

"Miriam" is a young lady who gave me such an opportunity. She sustained significant injury to her arm when a heavy counter top fell on her. She had severe problems with pain and an inability to move her arm well. Miriam had substantial ligament injury to her hand and thumb and a yanking injury to the entire arm resulting in nerve problems at the lower arm and also at the neck and thoracic outlet. She had a continued downhill course with respect to her symptoms. Her work life fell apart and her personal life as well took a significant downhill turn.

One of her major concerns, as is common with many of my patients, was she would not be able to hold her child when he was born. In fact, one of the more touching moments in my entire career was the day her son came in with her for her sixth month post-op checkup. Although I had known him since birth, he kept quite a distance from me. He knew me as the one who told his mom she couldn't lift him and hold him. During this particular visit, Miriam asked me if I would give her son the good news. I told him at this time she was able to lift and hold him again. I got one of the warmest hugs I've ever received from a young child.

Conversely, I have had unfortunate but inevitable experiences with patients who have not gotten better. Even when all is done in the appropriate manner, there are people who do not improve or who even get worse. These are the factors that give me not just the right to talk about conservative treatment but further the impetus to favor it as the first option. The hallmark of treatment in the prevention of nerve problems is to take the patient out of the offending environment which is causing the problem. For example, if you are a computer operator keying eight hours a day for five days a week and develop a problem, the answer seems clear. Alternative, less stressful keying styles, ergonomically improving your workstation, and frequent breaks to rest your hands are often helpful.

This brings to mind an old joke: A pediatrician walks into a room and her patient is banging his head against the wall. She says, "Johnny, why are you doing that?" Johnny stops, thinks a moment, and wisely replies, "Because if feels so good when I stop."

Just stop the activity causing the problem and the problem will often go away!

Conservative care is highly effective in treating nerve problems and especially carpal tunnel problems. When we get a patient early on and there is no severe scarring about the nerves or there are not nerves involved at multiple levels, conservative care is highly effective. In fact, we have found 50 percent of patients who come to us with an isolated carpal tunnel problem respond to conservative treatment and lifestyle modification. They never require surgery. Often a change in environment and a simple wrist splint used at night in conjunction with therapy are all that is required.

A conservative treatment program must be tailored to the individual and both patient and physician must understand the nature of the patient's complaints and symptoms. Therapy, when done appropriately, should not hurt and should never exacerbate or increase the symptoms.

Therapy is frequently helpful in the form of modalities such as cold, heat, and deep-heat delivery systems. They should be applied to the appropriate areas and often treatment needs to be applied at the neck and shoulder level as well as lower arm and carpal tunnel. Where the patient hurts, the patient should be treated.

Hot packs, ultrasound, and other heat modalities work by heating the tissues, softening scar tissue, and increasing circulation and nutrition to tissues and nerves. The increased blood flow allows excess fluid to be drained from the area. Cold modalities work by decreasing spasm and tissue irritability. The decrease in overall blood flow allows a lessening of fluid exudate entering the tissues and decreases swelling in this manner. The controversy of heat versus cold is one that has a straightforward answer, that is, apply ice in an acute injury for 24 hours then heat or ice thereafter, whichever feels better to the patient.

Transcutaneous Electrical Nerve Stimulation (TENS)/Acupuncture

TENS units are also helpful in many cases in calming down nerve symptoms. These work by actually stimulating the nerves to the point of exhaustion, thereby decreasing muscle spasm and the amount of intensity of nerve symptomatology. Acupuncture is believed to work in a similar manner and can be helpful as a modality if applied by a well-trained and qualified practitioner.

Massage

Massage is another form of therapy and treatment helpful for many patients. It works on the basis of increasing blood flow to a local area and also decreasing muscle spasm, which lessens the amount of compression on nerves. There are many forms of massage available today, and it is imperative the therapist performing this is a qualified therapist who understands the appropriate use of massage. Again, this should never hurt when being applied.

"Ed" is an interesting man who, early on, was a successful businessman. He developed problems with asbestosis and it was recommended he leave the indoor life and pursue outdoor activities to save his lungs. He took this to heart and became a deep sea fisherman. He worked for some time in this vocation and his lungs cleared nicely. Unfortunately, his work scaling fish was highly repetitive, and he injured his hands and elbow. He had some contact with *shiatsu* (a hands-on application combining acupressure [pressure points] and massage; related to acupuncture but without the use of needles) and found this quite helpful in treating these problems. Between his treatments and ours, he greatly improved—without surgery.

Ed saw another opportunity to move forward and pursued a career and eventually earned his credentials as a *shiatsu* therapist. He has essentially healed himself with respect to his injuries by using not only his own personal life experience but also the training he obtained in getting his license as a *shiatsu* therapist. Walt has a wonderful ability to adapt to life circumstances. With his injury, he realized he was not able to perform aggressive massage on a regular basis. He adapted his *shiatsu* training and style. He works more with people's emotional involvement and uses relaxation techniques and deep breathing exercises to help stabilize his patients.

Biofeedback/Meditation

Biofeedback and pain management approaches through relaxation techniques are often quite helpful. This may be in the form of a formalized biofeedback program, yoga, or activities such as *tai chi*, which is a martial art described as "meditation in motion." We have found these to be quite helpful in many patients in decreasing muscle spasm, stress, and ultimately pain.

Manipulation

They say you get what you pay for, but in this circumstance it appears you could be getting a bit more.

Spinal adjustments in the way of osteopathic treatments and chiropractic manipulation are helpful to many patients. These can be on the basis of soft tissue treatments as well as muscle energy or muscle exhausting techniques or actual spinal re-alignments and adjustments. It is imperative to be sure there is no underlying bone problem or significant ligament problem that would contraindicate these types of treatments. A complete medical workup as well as radiographic evaluation in the way of X-rays and MRIs when indicated should be done prior to undergoing any aggressive manipulation techniques. In the appropriate setting with an appropriately trained practitioner of joint and/or spinal manipulation, these two can be very helpful modalities.

Splints

In many cases, a splint used judiciously is helpful in calming down nerve problems. Splints are best used at night when the rest of the arm is not stressed by being used abnormally due to the restrictions of the splint. Often eight hours of splinting at night will help calm down tendinitis or inflammation enough to give a patient relief and eliminate most of the symptoms. Occasionally, I recommend the use of semi-rigid splints during the day when the arm is not being used aggressively.

There are some times, however, when splints can become significant issues and even result in some marital discord. Some of the splints we use are rather large and bulky and require the wearer to take up more room than usual. They are also hard and if someone is an active sleeper, assaulting a mate unknowingly can a source of some discord.

"Jim" had a significant ulnar nerve problem at his elbow. He got great relief by wearing a long-arm elbow splint every night to bed. As long as he continued to use the splint at night, Jim's nerve symptoms were calm, and he did not require any aggressive treatment or surgery. He did, though, have a significant nerve problem. We all had concern that at some point in time he would require surgery. Whenever he attempted to go a few nights without the splint, he had significantly increased symptoms.

Jim often came in alone to his office visits and we chatted a good deal about his business as well as life in general. On one particular occasion, his wife came in with him. A very sweet woman, she surprised us both when she gave both Jim and me an ultimatum: She made it clear, in no uncertain terms, she had reached her limit with respect to sleeping with the splint. She informed Jim unless he decided to go ahead with surgery and be rid of the splint, she would see that it was permanently implanted in his bowels. He quickly made a decision to have surgery to save the marriage and his dignity. Jim did wonderfully with surgery and quickly destroyed his splint.

Although I am a strong advocate of conservative care, there is a point at which splints may be more risky than the disease process and surgery itself!

The major disadvantage of splints is they cause patients to use their arms abnormally. The splinted wrist cannot be flexed or extended (bent up or down). In order to perform regular activities on any routine basis, the patient must compensate for these motions by abnormal use of other joints. When the wrist is splinted and a patient performs repetitive activities at work, the elbow and upper arm are stressed. This, over time, develops into a true cumulative trauma disorder or abnormal use syndrome. The patient experiences pain and symptoms at more than one level—a much more difficult problem to treat.

Repetitively stressing the outer aspect of the elbow results in problems such as a tennis elbow (tendinitis). If the medial (inner) side of the elbow is involved, the ulnar nerve is repetitively traumatized. This can result in ulnar nerve problems at the elbow (an additional nerve involved in the arm) and pain as well as numbness in the fourth and fifth digits.

When the elbow begins to hurt, patients may "splint" their actions themselves by not bending or straightening the elbow much as previously. Then they begin to overutilize the upper arm or shoulder area. The nerves at the neck and brachial plexus level (thoracic outlet) become involved by being pulled and inflamed on a regular basis. The shoulder joint itself also will often become involved at this point in time. The end result is what is then an abnormal use syndrome, hence, a cumulative trauma disorder. What was initially a simple problem starting at the wrist level now becomes a complex painful issue involving the entire arm.

It is easy to see how a person can become significantly disabled simply by attempting to continue an activity and ignoring its causative relationship to the problem. Further, by attempting to use the arm in an abnormal way, much more significant and difficult problems can result. Splinting at night will help calm down the tendinitis and may indeed help decrease the symptomatology. On the other hand, splints do not cure the problem, they simply help calm down the symptoms.

One patient comes to mind whenever I think about weaning patients from their splints. A pretty woman, with a speech impediment that caused her to stutter, had a severe injury requiring a number of different splints and contraptions over the course of many months. One of the splints had wires and rubber bands coming off at all angles. It was quite hideous to look and at, not to mention difficult to dress with. She spent a good deal of time in this splint, and I was quite excited the day of her visit when I could tell her she did not have to wear it anymore.

To my surprise and shock, when I told her she was free of her splint, she looked at me sadly. I asked what the problem was. She explained although the splint was truly unsightly, it was quite a help to her. She went on to say because of her speech impediment, one of her major problems was in meeting young men. She related since she had the splint on, whenever she was out in a public place, people would come over and begin talking to her. The splint was a wonderful conversation piece. She had met more new friends since she had the splint than ever in her life.

We came to a compromise. Medically, she really needed to come out of the splint and begin using her hand more regularly. I told her when she was going out somewhere and looking to meet people, she could wear the splint but otherwise the splint had to go. She was happy with this and moved on with her treatment and had a wonderful long-term result.

A final word about splints. Many patients come to us and have attempted conservative care with splints. These are often store-bought splints and the "one-size-fits-none" variety. It is important to remember a splint that is inappropriate or maintains the wrist or arm in an abnormal position is not helpful and may be harmful. It should be further understood that maintaining a wrist in a cocked-up position (extension) may be as harmful as maintaining it bent down (flexed) and can reproduce symptoms. Just because a store-bought splint does not help does not indicate splinting will not help, but rather the position may be incorrect. Splints that are custom-made and molded to a specific patient have the best chance of giving good relief.

In today's environment with "managed care" becoming more and more prevalent, the need to understand the concepts set forth here is even greater. One of our long-term staff members, Rachael, had an interesting conversation with an insurance adjustor some time ago. We were having trouble getting them to understand the concept of conservative care for carpal tunnel problems. They, in fact, were confused to the point where they stated they would not pay to have the patient get a splint but yet would pay for surgery. They further went on to tell us they had a new rule stating unless the patient had conservative care and splinting first, they would not be allowed to have surgery.

Rachael contacted the insurance representatives and explained to them we always attempted conservative care and splinting prior to considering any operative intervention. She further queried as to how we could possibly follow their protocol when they denied the use of splints. We eventually got around this and resolved the issue by making them aware of the fact 50 percent of our people did get better without the surgery. They agreed to let us go ahead with our conservative approach but really never quite understood we needed the splints to do it. This is unfortunately a common problem today. Many patients are never given the option of conservative care prior to being advised to have surgical treatment.

Medications and Injections

Prior to considering surgical intervention, if therapy and splints are not helpful, medications may be added. As you understand at this point in time, inflammation is a significant factor in causing median nerve and carpal tunnel problems. Often the use of an anti-inflammatory medication in the way of aspirin or one of the nonsteroidal anti-inflammatory drugs (NSAIDs) such as Motrin, Advil, Naprosyn, Clinoril, Feldene, or the like may help calm down the inflammation enough to decrease the patient's symptoms. I am not an advocate of long-term use of anti-inflammatory medications, but short-term use for intermittent episodes is often helpful in decreasing inflammation and may bring about early reversal of the inflammatory process.

Caution should be used with any of these medications. Short-term intermittent use or long-term use in problems such as severe arthritis is sometimes indicated. With long-term use, these medications have significant possible side effects in the way of liver and kidney damage. Ulcer disease and gastritis is not an unusual occurrence with these medications and, in fact, is rather common. With long-term use, it is rather inevitable people will generally begin to have some problems. Anti-inflammatory drugs, therefore, are best held for times when inflammation is acute and can be calmed down by a short course of the medication.

Speaking of ulcers, one of my patients is a very successful business entrepreneur. His job is essentially to straighten out companies that are having problems at the executive level. I made a quip to him one day that his job must be very stressful and this is exactly the kind of job that results in long-term stress problems such as heart disease and ulcers. Without batting an eye, he made the following statement: "I don't get ulcers, I give them."

What he meant was if you have a choice between pouring further stress on yourself or turning the stress outward, it's obviously better to do the latter. This, of course, should be with the limit that it should not hurt another individual when you do so. Stress is a significant component in disease and if we have ways to release our stress or at least re-direct it, we can often avoid its unpleasant effects. Stress, no doubt, increases nerve pain and personal pain in many ways, both physiologically and psychologically.

Nerve blocks by way of a test injection and the installation of cortisone at the carpal tunnel will allow for decreasing inflammation in the carpal tunnel. I almost always insist a patient try an injection once before considering operative intervention. If a patient gets temporary relief or at least a reduction of nerve symptoms and pain with a trial injection, from either the lidocaine or the cortisone, then he or she has a predictably better prognosis for relief with the surgery. If, however, the injection gives absolutely no relief to the patient, there is a poorer prognosis for improvement with surgical intervention. This certainly is not a 100-percent predictor but is helpful in making a decision as to whether to continue treating conservatively or more aggressively. A poor response may also indicate the major nerve problem may be at a different level and further evaluation may be necessary.

A word of caution about serial (multiple) injections in the carpal canal: If a patient gets only minimal, temporary relief with an injection, serial injections can cause problems. No more than two or three injections should be performed within the space of a year. If a patient does require multiple or serial injections, it is generally accepted to consider alternative treatments.

Unfortunately, there is a great deal of controversy among the medical community as to how to treat nerve problems today. There are many factors to consider in our patients' lives and also for their employers. It is often not "practical" to discontinue the activities causing the employees' problems. Finances are not the least of everyone's worries today. Single mothers, sole family providers, and others many times have no choice but to continue to try and work. At times, employers and even physicians who do not acknowledge or understand the nature of the problem may hinder the healing process.

"Sally" is an artist who worked for a number of years designing sweaters and clothes. Her working conditions were unfortunately quite difficult, not much better than a sweat-shop. She spent up to 14 hours at a time drawing and coloring designs in a hunched position. She developed significant problems with her arms and neck and reached a point of significant disability. She wasn't even able to hold a pen very well. Drawing or even sitting in the posture of drawing caused her severe pain.

Sally went to her boss but was told nothing could be done. She sought medical treatment and was unable to obtain any good relief. She realized she had a substantial problem and even though she was told there was nothing that could be done, she came to realize her life situation was becoming intolerable.

She sought treatment from a number of directions. She began therapy and learned relaxation techniques. Medications were somewhat helpful. Her nerve studies showed significant pathologic involvement but even with this, Sally was not dissuaded from moving forward.

During the course of her treatment, Sally sought multiple alternative treatments including cranio-sacral therapy, which is manipulation of the joints of the skull. This was quite helpful for her headaches and she also got good relief from a support group for people who were going through significant life changes.

Sally has continued to do well and improve. In spite of markedly positive nerve studies and injury, she has excellent relief from pain through her ability to adapt and modify her lifestyle within the limitations of her disease. She is now drawing, although not in a sweatshop environment. She is one of our success stories and has gone on to help others by teaching them as she did herself.

Suffice it to say, at this point the limitations of conservative care and treatment are bound only by the imagination. There are many alternative treatment options available today. What is important to realize at this time is conservative treatment of nerve problems does work and is often successful. Many patients get better without ever taking that trip to the operating room and go on to lead normal lives. Remember, the decision to have surgery should be your choice and at least a trial of conservative care prior to proceeding with surgery should be given to almost everyone.

Surgery—Who Should Have It? When and Why?

CHAPTER 8

Surgery, like many things in life, is not for everyone! I start this chapter with this statement because there are no truer words or more helpful advice that can be spoken to any patient by a surgeon. When surgery is right, it is the best thing that could ever happen. When it is wrong, it can be both a patient's and a surgeon's worst nightmare. I often tell my patients surgery is like marriage. When it's with the right person at the right time, it's great. On the other hand, if it's not right, it can be a catastrophe. The key to successful surgery is a realistic understanding of the patient's problem, symptoms and complaints, and a realistic expectation by the physician and patient as to the outcome from the surgery.

"Carol" found this out the hard way. She had been told by her initial surgeon she had carpal tunnel, could have surgery, and go back to her job at a pill manufacturing plant almost immediately after the surgery. She was told the surgery was "no big deal" and assured there would be no problems, and her hand would be normal again post-operatively.

This could not have been further from reality. Unfortunately, Carol was sent back to work very soon after her surgery.

She had progressive problems with pain, swelling, numbness, and tingling in her hand and arm. Not only did she *not* improve from the surgery; she got worse. Her life became a nightmare and she was repeatedly told the surgery was "fine." She developed a full-blown reflex sympathetic dystrophy (RSD). Her arm became more painful, stiff, numb, and useless. This happens to approximately one in a few hundred patients and we really don't know why. Instead of having mild pain from a simple trauma such as surgery or an injury such as a broken wrist, these patients develop severe pain, swelling, and disability. Their hands actually swell and change color, and the hair on the arm darkens and changes in texture. Severe pain is the cardinal and overwhelming complaint. The key to treating this problem is early recognition of the symptoms and therapy. Intensive therapy and proper medications early on generally will calm down this complex but many times the patients are left with significant residual effects. Unfortunately, the RSD was not recognized in Carol and the treating physician just told her to keep on using her hand and continue to work.

By the time Carol got to us, she had a severe case of RSD and her entire arm was significantly disabled. She required intensive therapy and subsequently repeat surgery. Carol had some relief but her hand has never become normal. We were fortunate to be able to get Carol to a point where she feels the pain in the arm is tolerable. Carol relates that although she is not able to use the arm for many daily activities, she is at least able to enjoy life. She controls her pain via biofeedback and pain management techniques. Thanks to her strong will, Carol is approaching a more normal life at this point; however, she is not capable of returning to her previous activities and has never achieved the unrealistic result promised by her initial treating doctor. Carol is indeed someone who taught me as well as many of my other patients that surgery is not always what we expect it to be and many times we are better off without it.

We have come a long way with medicine but we are still nowhere near understanding why many treatments do and do not work. Certainly, technology has advanced and our surgical procedures are done more deftly and successfully. Conversely, patients come into my office every day with problems for which we have no cures. I am still at times depressed and embarrassed at the limited knowledge we have.

When surgeons meet and discuss surgeries, why some operations work and some don't, heated discussions often arise. Theories, ideas, and explanations abound. Unfortunately, the bottom line answer is we really just don't know. I often joke when explaining surgical procedures and say we simply act as mechanics and realign the tissues; then God heals them!

Unfortunately, we are not mechanics. We are physicians and deal with the most complex and yet magnificent machine known—the human body. Each person reacts differently to the same surgical procedures. Although there are some predictors and some relative regularities with certain operations and their outcomes, we never know with certainty how a surgery is going to turn out. Even in the same person, when I operate on one hand and then the other, I cannot predict each outcome. Patients often tell me although one hand did great, the other is not quite as good or is different.

A person who comes to mind is "Molly." I operated on her right hand for a median nerve problem and she had all kinds of post-operative problems. She developed many symptoms of reflex sympathetic dystrophy and significant discomfort and stiffness in the arm. We went through a prolonged course of therapy and avoided any significant problems. She finally did achieve good relief from the surgery, but this took months. When she came into the operating room for the surgery on her other hand, she looked me straight in the eye and asked, "Is this one going to work?" As you can imagine, this gave me less than a great feeling of confidence. My self-esteem, ego, and energy level, were lowered quite a few notches. I even began to question whether we were right diagnostically in her case. To my great relief, she woke up from the surgery in the recovery room and told me this one was different. And in fact, it was! She has experienced excellent relief with the second hand and none of the symptoms or reactivity she had in the other arm. She has been pain-free from day one although she had the same genetics, the same capacity to heal, and the same disease in both arms, one hand had significant problems and the second none whatsoever. I have seen the opposite as well where the first hand did well and the second had difficulty. The explanation remains a mystery.

These reactions and outcomes are not uncommon in surgery. Each operation is a unique event! This is an important point to be pondered as well as remembered for any patient who is thinking about elective surgery, even those patients with prior personal experience.

The decision as to who should have carpal tunnel surgery and when should be based on one and only one factor: what the patient decides. I cannot emphasize too strongly the role of a physician is to educate his or her patients. If you as a patient understand the underlying pathophysiology and nature of your disease, then you can make rational decisions as to what type of treatment you need. You can further educate us as physicians to the best decision and direction for you. Ultimately, you can decide on the right treatment for yourself be it surgical or nonsurgical.

I often find my most obstinate patients who initially protest even the concept of surgery become my best surgical results. These are generally people who have strong wills and a strong desire to heal themselves without any help or outside interference. "Amanda" comes to mind as such an individual. Her husband, "Ken," was a patient of mine for some time and told me during a visit his wife was quite symptomatic with numbness and tingling in her arms. He told me she had made it perfectly clear to him she would "never have surgery." I told him certainly this was a reasonable way to think but at least she should give herself the benefit of understanding her problem.

Amanda ultimately did come in for an evaluation and turned out to be a delightful lady who is not only strong-willed but wonderfully capable of understanding her problems. She was indeed adamantly opposed to any surgery. Amanda undertook treatment with us and ultimately told me she had to have surgery. When I confronted her with the fact she had told both her husband and me she never would have surgery, she related her issue was more of control than surgery. As long as this was *her* decision, she was fine with surgery. The key here was that Amanda maintained control of her body and her life. Amanda has had more than one operation and in fact has gone on to have thoracic outlet surgery, which is about as risky a venture as you can undertake with regard to nerve surgery in the upper extremities. She's had a wonderful recovery and has improved greatly from her previous status. Although she still has some low-level symptoms, Amanda is at this point leading a relatively normal life. Through understanding her disease, she has made intelligent decisions and helped to dictate her care through three surgeries with good relief from her pain. She understood why and when she needed each intervention and also made choices based on her own intuitive understanding of her body, her symptoms, and her personal needs.

Dr. Bernie Siegel relates a wonderful story in one of his writings in which he talks about a small boy who was in the hospital for cancer. To empower the young boy with some control over his care and in essence his life, he is given a pad and some crayons. The hospital is very busy and many people come in to examine the young man. Any doctor who wishes to examine this child is given the task of drawing a picture. It is further understood unless the doctor is willing to draw a picture for the young boy, he or she does not get the privilege of examining him.

This points out a basic issue in any care. This young man could obviously not grasp some of the concepts of the intimate details of his disease, but he certainly was capable of understanding the relationship between a patient and physician should be one of give and take. If the doctors were not willing to give, he certainly would not let them take from him, be it even an examination. The concept of patients in pain versus patients with cancer is not a quantum leap. A relationship and mutual respect must exist if intelligent and rational treatment plans are to be born.

Before contemplating any surgery or surgical intervention, a definite sequence of events should take place. First and most important, you need to develop a relationship with the surgeon you choose. This should be a person with whom you are able to talk! As a patient you must feel free to discuss motivations, goals, fears, and long-term desires. Your surgeon should communicate a sense he or she understands you and your disease. There must be open communication so this person understands just what it is that bothers you.

I remember early in my career sitting in an exam room with a large gentleman. He was accompanied by a woman and had come in for a hand problem no one seemed to be able to help him with. I took a detailed history and had a fairly good idea of what was going on with the hand. It seemed to me a rather straightforward problem, and I wondered why no one had been able to help him with it.

I told him I wished to examine him and move my stool closer. I reached out for his hand and the woman said, "Don't!" I sat back in my chair and stopped for a moment. I then went to reach forward again and was met by the same cry, "Don't!" At this point, I rolled my stool back a few inches and turned to the lady who was with him. I asked why she kept saying "Don't!" every time I went to reach for his hand.

She said, "I wasn't talking to you, I was talking to him." I queried further and she explained he had cold-cocked the last two doctors who tried to examine him as soon as they touched his arm.

I informed them both I thought I'd have as difficult a time as the other doctors in helping him. We treated him based on history rather than a detailed examination.

To be fair, not all surgeons are great communicators. I know some wonderful surgeons who can't even relate to their own families. As long as you feel your surgeon understands your needs, then you have a good start. You must, however, be able to obtain a good understanding of your disease and your options. If these two key ingredients are present, you are on your way to healing.

Before undertaking any surgical intervention, with the exception of life or limb-threatening disease, all conservative measures should be tried. These may include taking the patient out of the offending environment (such as a job that is causing the problem) or at least modifying the use of the patient's hands and arms. Medications may be tried on a short-term basis but should not be depended on in the long-term. Splints and therapy are also quite helpful as previously discussed.

This brings to mind a patient named "Gus," who was very upset when he came to our center. He had been treated by another physician and told he had a nerve problem at the wrist. He began treatment and the doctor operated on his elbow for a secondary issue with no explanation. Post-operatively, he really wasn't able to move his arm freely and was in severe pain. His arm became increasingly stiff and rigid. His elbow was worse, which he believed was a direct result of the surgery that had not helped his pain at all. It took us a while to come to an agreement for treatment with which we were both comfortable. I agreed to perform further surgery on him where he thought the problem was if all conservative measures failed. In return for this, he agreed to try our conservative therapy program and learn more about his illness.

I was unsure if he would keep his part of the bargain, but he stayed with us—partly because we believed in him and frankly because no one else would take his case. The interesting fact is that although his electrical studies were negative and all signs pointed to the fact he should not get better with surgery, he knew exactly where his problem was. Although outwardly he appeared to be an enraged young man, he really did understand his disease better than any of us. He had the surgery and when he awoke from the operation, he told me his pain was gone. He went on to finish the therapy program and resumed a normal life without any pain. His anger was simply frustration at the fact we as a medical society could not understand him and his problems. He was certainly not one of my easier patients but indeed one of the more rewarding.

I want at this time to make a point about therapy. Most therapists have good intentions, but therapy can be a double-edged sword. There are many schools of thought as to how to treat pain problems and nerve injuries. A key factor to remember is whatever the treatment, it should not hurt! When performed by therapists who understand your disease and your problem, therapy should feel good. Therapy should calm symptoms down and make you feel better. The "no pain, no gain" theory is exactly that—a theory. Treatment, except in very rare circumstances, should not be uncomfortable at all and should help to alleviate symptoms. At times therapy, like surgery, makes people worse. You as the patient must understand your disease so you can guide both your physicians and your therapists. Remember, pain is a signal something is wrong.

Injections are helpful at times and when used judiciously on an occasional basis can relieve symptoms and avoid the need for operations. Multiple and serial injections should generally be avoided.

When, then, is it time to have surgery? Again I repeat: When you feel all other avenues have been exhausted and the symptoms are unlivable and interfering significantly with your life. Of course, determining exactly when symptoms are significantly interfering with your life is not always an easy decision.

I remember an 86-year-old gentleman who came to me with a request to have carpal tunnel surgery that week. I asked him to tell me a bit about himself and his history. He told me this was not necessary; he just wanted to have the surgery because he had a positive EMG. I explained to him almost everyone in his age group has a positive EMG for carpal tunnel and this doesn't necessarily mean he needed surgery. I further explained to him the results of his examination were fairly benign, he had no muscle wasting, and he did not have constant or persistent numbness. (I also told him the arthritis in his neck was significant, and I did not believe the hand surgery would give him what he wanted.) He told me his lifestyle was being dramatically altered and he absolutely needed the surgery. He explained he played tennis four days a week and went to the gym and lifted weights three days a week. His forehand was just not as strong as it used to be. This was bothersome to him and he wished to have the surgery to fix these concerns.

This is in sharp contrast to another gentleman patient who presented a swollen hand, numbness, tingling, and complete loss of use of his hand for any functions. He was unable to feed himself or dress in the morning due to his severe pain, discomfort, and swelling. He, too, was in his mid-eighties but was in my opinion a candidate for surgery, and we proceeded the following week. His result was excellent and he was able to go back to routine daily activities. To my knowledge, he has not taken up tennis or weight lifting, and perhaps if he did, he would tell me my operation didn't work.

These are two patients with requests for the same operation but for very different reasons. I, as a surgeon, had the difficult choice of saying yes to one and no to the other. Although I tried to educate the first man on the realistic expectations for the surgery, he was not willing to hear these. Perhaps he was right and I did him a disservice. On the other hand, in making a judgment, I told him I could not in good conscience go ahead with surgery that could leave him worse than he was at the time. The possibility of a tender scar and a weaker grip from the surgery could, indeed, have altered his lifestyle much more significantly than he was aware. A better choice would have been to try and modify his workout schedule and try conservative treatment first. If he then continued to worsen, surgery could be considered once he understood the realistic goals.

When considering surgery, you must understand the nature of the operation and its possible risks, and these should be explained to you in detail. Every surgery that has benefits also has possible problems or complications. If you understand these clearly before proceeding, the choices will be more obvious.

Ask what you can expect from the operation and what you will realistically be able to do—6, 12, and 24 weeks postoperatively.

"Isaac," aged 72, was having some problems with his golf game. He had a disease called Dupuytrens in which the tissues of the palm contract, not allowing straightening of the fingers. Surgery is performed to allow better opening of the hand. Dupuytrens is a difficult problem in that patients generally have no pain and no significant disability. There are significant possible complications with Dupuytrens surgery including the possibility of damage to nerves and blood vessels as well as reflex sympathetic dystrophy. In his case, Isaac was concerned he was not able to get his hand around his golf club. He saw a surgeon who performed surgery for removal of this fixed scar tissue in the palm.

Isaac was one of the unfortunate individuals who developed reflex sympathetic dystrophy. He also had a complication from the nerve block at his neck. He developed a reflex sympathetic dystrophy with significant pain, swelling, and discomfort in the hand as well as stiffness. He also acquired a significant ulnar nerve problem in the arm with severe compromise in ulnar nerve function. He has had substantial problems with muscle wasting and an inability to use his hand for any fine motor activities.

Isaac decided to proceed conservatively rather than have further surgery to try and alleviate his pain. He is a strong individual who has good personal motivation. He felt further surgery could cause him as much harm as good. The options in either direction are reasonable. He has made some real life decisions, accepting certain long-term disabilities as compared to the possible risks. His major regret is that he had surgery in the first place and developed problems that could not be foreseen.

You should be aware of the risk of recurrence of your disease. It is well known that going back to the same type of activity that caused the problem initially can result in recurrence of disease. Recurrent scarring about nerves is a serious problem and some reports relate up to 30 percent of people who have carpal tunnel surgery have recurrence of disease. This incidence of recurrence can be decreased by taking proper precautions and treating the hand "nicely" post-operatively.

Many surgeons don't follow their patients for more than four to six weeks post-op. They actually have no idea as to whether the problem recurs or goes away once patients resume normal activities. I have found many patients continue to have symptoms but think these are "normal" and "to be expected."

Remember the following points when considering surgery:

1. The decision to have or not to have surgery, except in emergency circumstances, should be yours as the patient and yours alone.

2. The major function of your surgeon is to educate you about your disease and the nature of the process. He or she should also educate you as to each of your options and the benefits and also risks of each of these.

3. Therapy, splints, medications, and injections should always be tried before surgical intervention is entertained.

4. Trust your own feelings.

5. When all else fails, surgery is an option as long as it is a mutual decision made by you and your surgeon, and you are comfortable that you understand why it is being done and what to expect from the surgery.

6. Be realistic about your expectations from the surgery before proceeding.

Although there is certainly no exact formula for determining the appropriate time to proceed with surgery, the above guidelines can at least make the decision easier. There are, of course, situations where surgery must be done but these are usually fairly obvious and the decisions usually fairly easy to make when you as the patient understand the exact nature of the problem.

Let's Talk Surgery

CHAPTER 9

As you now understand, carpal tunnel symptoms develop when there is progressive swelling inside the carpal canal. This puts increased pressure on the nerve and over the course of time with the formation of more scar tissue, less and less stress and pressure are required to produce the nerve symptoms. Once the issue becomes permanent in nature and therapy, splints, medications, and injections are not helpful, it is reasonable to consider surgical intervention. The obvious question you should be asking at this point is: "Is this fixable?"

The answer to this question is *yes* and *no*. Surgery can often relieve the symptoms associated with carpal tunnel problems and there are many people who get relief from the surgery. The question we really need to ask is whether we've made these hands normal.

My dad tells a wonderful story about a pocket knife found lying on the street. This is a beautiful piece made of solid brass and stainless steel with fine etchings and carvings on it. In and of itself, this knife is an inanimate object not capable of any independent activities. If a collector finds this knife, he might well polish it and place it in a display case. He would then wonder who owned it previously and conjecture about their stories. Was there a history of happiness, tragedy, fame, or fortune?

A sculptor might find this knife and create a beautiful work of art.

The knife could be found by a young boy who would have hours of enjoyment whittling a piece of wood and studying its etchings.

A thief might come upon it and use our inanimate friend as an instrument of destruction, wielding it to steal or even murder.

A surgeon might find this knife, pocket it, and one day use it to save someone's life by performing an emergency tracheotomy where no other instruments were available.

Remember, surgery does entail the use of knives. It is vital we remember every person who owns a knife or scalpel does not use it in the appropriate or exact manner which was intended originally. Take care in choosing your surgeon. Be sure he or she has only your best interest in mind. You must feel confident your surgeon is truly a healer by your judgment of him or her as a person.

Although symptom relief is common with carpal tunnel surgery, there are a number of patients who have recurrent problems. Most patients modify the way they use their hands and arms after they have surgery. Although the severe symptoms are often improved, there are still minor issues that remain in many patients, especially those with long-standing nerve problems. Many patients still have residual numbness and tingling and altered sensibility. In many cases surgery is indeed helpful. However, we should not confuse this with making the hand "normal."

Whenever surgical intervention is performed, scar tissue is removed and scar tissue is created. Any insult to the body, be it a gunshot or a surgical incision, results in the body forming scar tissue. As we discussed before, treating the surgical wound

112

and arm nicely after the surgery is definitely helpful in decreasing the amount of aggressive scar that re-forms but nonetheless scar always does form after surgical intervention. Understanding this, we can see surgery may help the situation, but we should not expect it to make the situation normal. When it comes close to normal, then we are way ahead of the game. However, there is no way to tell who will get an optimal result and who will not.

"Sam" came to me with severe pain in his arm. He had progressive disability with respect to use of his arm, which was getting worse over the course of time. He had already had two surgeries at his elbow for his ulnar nerve and related that in spite of these, his pain continued to increase. He had a minor insult after his second surgery and was unable to use the arm at all. He was definitely a person who had not gotten better with surgical intervention. He told me his only desire was to be able to throw a ball again with his children. He realized this might never be possible, but felt his arm was not tolerable in its current state.

We did undertake repeat surgery for Sam with relocation of his ulnar nerve at the elbow. He had an extraordinarily prolonged recovery time as we expected, due to the severe damage we found in the nerve. In fact, due to his two previous surgeries and the severe scarring that formed about the nerve, there were portions that were so frayed and tattered, I questioned myself whether the nerve would ever function normally.

Through sheer determination and will, Sam continued with the post-operative program. It took us six months but one day he walked in and said, "Scott, I'm glad I had the surgery." I knew we had made a breakthrough at that point. By the year mark, he indeed was throwing a ball with his children. He succeeded due to an iron constitution and his understanding of the nature of his underlying nerve problem. This gave Sam the ability to keep moving and avoid significant recurrent scarring.

In some ways, Sam and I were lucky. There are absolutely times when it is appropriate to perform repeat surgery in spite of previous surgical failures. The decision to go ahead must be with absolute commitment on the part of both surgeon and patient, understanding there are indeed no guarantees with surgery.

With this said, there are a number of different surgical procedures performed to treat carpal tunnel problems. Each of them has its proponents but each also carries with it significant inherent risks. One of the key points I wish to make here is no surgery is risk-free. Any surgeon who tells you there is no risk to a surgery either has not performed enough surgeries or is naive about the possible complications. Each and every surgery carries with it a certain amount of risk, and you must be willing to accept that risk prior to proceeding with any operative intervention. Further, there are some risks of which patients are not made aware. With any surgery, there is the possibility of damage to nerves, tendons, blood vessels and ligament structures. There is also the risk of reflex sympathetic dystrophy.

"Rose" learned this the hard way. She saw a doctor for a small cyst on her finger and another at her wrist. She also had some mild intermittent symptoms of numbness and tingling. She was taken immediately to surgery without any further workup or therapy. Her surgery lasted eleven minutes, which is extraordinarily short. The surgeon performed a removal of the cysts from her finger and wrist, and a carpal tunnel release. Unfortunately, along with this, the radial artery was cut in the forearm and the nerves were inadvertently cut in the finger. Post-operatively, Rose had significantly increased symptoms of numbness, tingling, pain, and discomfort.

Rose subsequently came under our care and required an extensive amount of treatment in the way of therapy, splints, and further surgery to actually re-anastomose (connect) her cut nerves. She required long-term rehabilitation for close to a year just to reach a point of livability with her pain.

Rose has, at this time, gone back to a reasonably normal life, although her hand and arm are not normal. We've never quite been able to get her back to her status prior to surgeries. She is someone who learned the hard way surgery is not always what it's meant to be. She also learned it pays to get to know your surgeon and options prior to having surgery. She has overcome her pain by sheer will and good nature. Instead of anger at her situation, she focused on healing and did just that.

The point must be brought out once again; although surgery may be successful in relieving carpal tunnel symptoms, a patient who goes back to the same activity and environment that caused the problem initially is likely to develop symptoms once again. What most fail to understand, patients and doctors alike, is once surgery is necessary it is really too late to "fix the problem." At this point, we are just relieving the symptoms. The key to understanding successful surgery is the realization once an operation has been performed, the risk of recurrence of the same problem is markedly increased if the patient returns to the environment that caused the problem in the first place.

It is often desirable to leave the environment prior to having surgery. If all that is necessary is getting out of the job or situation which is causing the symptoms, then surgery may be avoided. It is imperative patients are not exposed post-operatively to the same traumas that caused the initial problem. When they are, many require repeat surgery, or worse, are not even candidates for a second procedure and have to live their lives in pain. Second-time surgery is even less predictable and rewarding than first-time surgery.

How Is Carpal Tunnel Surgery Done?

The basic common denominator in all carpal tunnel surgeries is releasing the transverse carpal ligament, which means cutting the ligament to make it less tense and rigid over the nerve and tendon structures in the carpal tunnel. This gives relief in many patients and at times is all that is required. In many cases, however, there is scar tissue surrounding and encasing the median nerve and its branches. Unless the nerve is freed from this scar tissue, many patients will remain with symptoms due to the fact that the nerve is bound down and not able to move well. This results in a persistent traction neuropathy with continued and at times progressive nerve complaints. These are often the patients who have unrecognized secondary levels of nerve involvement (such as at the neck or thoracic outlet levels).

I had an interesting experience that clarified how each of us views life differently. I was examining the X-ray of a youngster who had broken his collarbone. In order to take this X-ray the entire chest cavity is exposed on the X-ray film. The boy happened to be the son of a local cardiologist and we were looking at the films together.

Tom commented to me his son's heart and lungs looked good. I turned to Tom, stopping in the middle of my dictation. I realized I was so totally focused on the collarbone and ribs I didn't even notice the heart and lungs as part of the film. We all see best from our own perspective and point of view. As an orthopedic surgeon, I view X-rays as a tool for evaluating bone and joint problems. He, as a cardiologist, sees heart and lungs and really doesn't notice the bones. How interesting we approach issues from only one point of view. Blessed is the individual who can maintain an open mind.

It is easy to apply this to nerve problems. If doctors evaluate patients with pain and numbness by focusing only on carpal tunnel, what do you think will happen? The entire length of nerve from neck to brachial plexus through the forearm is not even considered. This is why many patients go undiagnosed and untreated even though they have significant nerve disease.

"Nadia" works in a paper manufacturing plant. Her job consists of repetitive wrist, hand, and arm motions with reaching, pulling, and pushing. She had significant problems with her arms and severe pain and discomfort for two years. She had seen a multitude of doctors and was given varied diagnoses from over-reactivity to "recurrent carpal tunnel problems." She was also diagnosed as having arthritis and a muscle inflammation disorder called fibromyalgia.

What was apparent by her history is she had progressive problems with pain and discomfort. She had severe pain she described as "like a knife" sticking into her left brachial plexus. She had problems on the right as well. Nadia described these symptoms as increasing with her increased workload and decreasing with decreased workload. She reached a point where she was unable to live with her pain but she had discomfort all the time. By the end of a 50-hour work week, she required three days just to calm her pain. She had significant headaches as well as the severe arm pain.

Nadia described a classic cumulative trauma disorder or repetitive motion syndrome. Although this was "entertained" by one or two doctors, she had been told there was nothing that could be done for her. The doctor who did her previous carpal tunnel surgery 15 years earlier told her it was impossible for her to have any recurrent problems with her carpal tunnel. He said there was nothing wrong and she should return to work.

This is a classic example of following a standard paradigm and seeing only from one point of view. Without looking further, no one was able to pin down her diagnosis. When we listened to her story, we heard a classic cumulative trauma problem.

She was smart enough to take herself out of the offending work environment. In a few short weeks, she noted a marked improvement. The only one who really knew where she was heading and where she should be going was the patient herself. From her employer's and doctors' points of view, the dogma stated she had been "fixed," so no one actually took the time to listen to the patient.

There are a number of ways to release the ligament today and multiple variations on how carpal tunnel surgery can be performed. There is no one ideal operation and some are poor. Following is a brief discussion on the benefits and possible problems with each operation.

Standard Open Carpal Tunnel Release

This procedure was popularized by Dr. Phalen in the 1950s. This is the "standard by which all other carpal tunnel operations are judged." Unfortunately, this operation gained popularity at a time when repetitive traumas and the type of problems we see today were not prevalent. In its time it was a good operation and generally enough to give people relief from their night pain and symptoms. It was mainly done on older individuals who did not require high demand of their hands and wrists.

The procedure is done by making an incision in the palm and exposing the ligament proper. A knife or scissor is then used to open the ligament and expose the median nerve. With this procedure, the surgeon has the option of fully freeing the median nerve and its branches if scar tissue is encountered and also cleaning out any inflamed tissue within the carpal tunnel such as tenosynovitis.

"Bethany" had carpal tunnel surgery done by a well-meaning surgeon. Release was obtained in the ligament and she got some mild but incomplete early relief post-op. Unfortunately, she was returned to her job seven days after surgery. As soon as she returned to work, she had the same symptoms of numbness, tingling, and pain radiating up the arm as she had pre-operatively. The longer she continued to work, the more severe and progressive her symptoms became. Within a matter of weeks, she was worse than she was before the surgery.

What Bethany failed to understand was although she'd had carpal tunnel surgery, she was not "cured." She was told by her doctor she'd had surgery so her problem was gone. He said her symptoms and pain must all be in her head.

Luckily, she sought further help and treatment. Once she got out of the offending work environment, her symptoms calmed down and improved. We have been able to reach a point of pain-free function in this arm. There is no doubt returning to the type of work and activities she performed previously is out of the question. Although surgery was "successful," it did not make this hand normal.

The open procedure definitely has the advantage of assuring complete release of the ligament. It also gives the advantage of ruling out any other covert type pathology such as tumors or other problems which may be present and are not readily diagnosed. The disadvantage of this procedure is the ligament is left open and the patient is not able to begin wrist flexion (bending the wrist down) for approximately two to three weeks until a new looser ligament begins to form. If the patient flexes the wrist, the possibility of subluxation (popping out) of the structures from the carpal tunnel is great. This could result in problems down the line and instability of the nerve and tendon structures in the carpal canal. The further disadvantage of this procedure is without the early motion and flexion at the wrist, the median nerve may rebind and scar down in that it is not moving or gliding early on after the procedure. Although this procedure has its limitations, this is the standard by which all others are judged.

119

Endoscopic Median Nerve Decompression

A popular form of carpal tunnel surgery today is the so-called endoscopic technique. There are a number of different approaches popular today using this technique incorporating either one or two portals (openings) in the skin. The operation incorporates a transverse incision at the wrist and exposure of the carpal tunnel at the wrist level. An arthroscope, which is a small telescope used to view the under surface of the ligament, is then placed inside of the carpal tunnel. Looking up from inside the carpal canal, the ligament is transected from within.

The advantage to this procedure is dissection is not carried out through the superficial layers of the palm and the palmar fascia, which is the superficial portion of the ligament. This requires much less surgical dissection and is reported to have a decreased amount of pain and discomfort post-operatively.

A major advantage of this operation is wrist motion can be started early on post-operatively in that the superficial fascia in the palm is not completely opened; therefore the danger of subluxation of the deep structures (the median nerve and flexor tendons) is not present. This also carries with it the advantage of less probability of post-operative pain in the palm at the incision site or so-called "pillar pain."

The disadvantage to the endoscopic technique is it is a highly demanding technique requiring extensive training to perfect. There are a number of different ways to perform endoscopic techniques and a significant amount of variation as how these techniques are performed. There is a substantial learning curve for the surgeon performing these techniques, which means until he or she has done quite a few, complications are likely. The possibility of laceration of the median nerve as well as palmar arch (the blood supply and circulation to the hand) is real with these procedures and has been reported. There is also the possibility of injury to the motor branch of the median nerve and the ulnar nerve secondary to improper placement of the instrumentation. The end result of these nerve injuries can be substantial in the way of numbness and dysfunction of the hand.

Another significant limitation of the standard technique of endoscopic carpal tunnel release is the median nerve itself cannot be viewed via the scope. It is therefore conceivable if there is significant scarring about the nerve or a significant amount of tendinitis or other pathology in the deep carpal canal, it can be missed by this procedure.

We perform a modification of this procedure in the appropriate patients, and this allows slightly larger incisions at the wrist and the hand level. After releasing the ligament via endoscopic technique, the carpal canal as well as the median nerve can be identified and evaluated. If there is significant inflammation about the flexor tendons, a synovectomy (cleaning out of the inflamed lining) can be performed at the same sitting. This is a compromise between the standard open technique and the closed endoscopic technique.

Mini-Incision (Blind) Techniques

There are some surgeons who perform a mini-incision technique touted as a minimal carpal tunnel release. This is a procedure where a small incision is made at the wrist and an instrument is passed beneath the ligament in a nonvisualized fashion and the transverse carpal ligament is blindly cut. The instrument itself is a knife and is passed beneath the transverse carpal ligament in a blind fashion. This procedure has all of the risks and possible complications described above with the endoscopic technique but more so because it is done without any visualization. It must be undertaken only with extreme caution and trepidation.

The second and most important danger with this procedure is a knife is being shoved blindly down through the carpal canal and the possibility of laceration to the digital nerves and specifically the motor branch is real. In approximately 3 to 5 percent of cases, the motor branch of the median nerve, which controls the thenar muscles, has a takeoff (originates) at the very ulnar or little finger side of the hand and then traverses into the thenar muscles of the thumb. If a blind procedure is performed, this motor branch can be transected (cut). If this happens, the function of the thenar musculature will cease. What this means is the patient will lose opposition of the thumb. Without the opposable thumb, the hand loses approximately 30 percent of its normal function. This is a procedure which, in my opinion, has risks unacceptable in view of other available surgical options.

"Sheena" came in after having had both hands operated on simultaneously with a mini-incision technique for carpal tunnel problems. Although she'd had both hands done, she never got any relief from her pain, discomfort, numbness, or tingling. When we discussed the situation, she informed me she'd had problems for some time and substantial numbness was awakening her at night. When she went back and told her surgeon she still had symptoms, she was told she was "crazy" and there was nothing more that could be done since surgery had been completed.

On further evaluation, her examination and nerve tests were markedly positive for residual significant disease. We subsequently performed open median nerve decompression and she has done well with good relief from her symptoms.

It is important to realize here when limited surgeries are performed, there is risk of either damage to nerve structures or incomplete release of the ligament. There are certainly many patients who have gotten relief with these "mini-procedures," but there are also quite a few walking around today who continue to have problems. Many suffer silently with their problems because they are told there is nothing else that can be done. If you have had surgery but still have symptoms, a search for the cause of those symptoms should not be abandoned.

Open Median Nerve Decompression with Transverse Carpal Ligament Reconstruction and Other "Salvage" Procedures

A relatively new procedure that is becoming more popular for patients with recurrent carpal tunnel or patients who have already had carpal tunnel surgery and "failed" is open decompression with reconstruction of the transverse carpal ligament. This has the advantages of the open median nerve surgery with full visualization of all structures in the carpal canal. It also carries the advantage of the endoscopic technique, which allows early mobilization with wrist flexion/extension. The procedure itself is much more extensive and generally reserved for patients who require repeat surgery for severe damage to the nerve. When necessary, neurolysis and tenosynovectomy can be performed. With reconstruction of the ligament, the patient is allowed to begin wrist motion and nerve gliding immediately post-operatively. We have found this a useful procedure for patients with severe disease or with recurrent carpal tunnel problems. Other surgeons may use a fat graft or muscle transfers to cover the nerve in recurrent cases. By allowing early motion of the wrist with early nerve gliding, we can often optimize post-operative results.

Laser Surgery

A popular misconception today is the laser can make carpal tunnel surgery easier. The laser is a relatively new tool used in some orthopaedic procedures but has not been effective in the carpal canal. The heat generated by the laser can be detrimental to the median nerve and can actually destroy it. The results of carpal tunnel laser surgeries I have seen have been little short of catastrophic. Currently the laser has no place in the carpal tunnel. Many people today confuse laser surgery with endoscopic surgery, which is the use of a light source but not a light-heat source.

"June" discovered this in the worst way possible. She had surgery done on both hands by a surgeon who was performing the endoscopic technique with the "laser." Her first hand was done via his standard endoscopic technique, and she got minimal, if any, relief. She continued to have problems with pain, numbness, and tingling. Her other hand was then done by the same surgeon and the ligament "released," or cut by laser. Unfortunately, the median nerve itself was lasered. It was burned, charred, and transected.

She underwent surgery for repair of the nerve but to this day sensation has never returned because of the severe thermal damage as well as transection. She has severe muscle wasting as well. Although we've treated her hand and arm for some time, she has never had return of normal function. We've at least been able to calm her pain, but she has never regained function. Her retrospective analysis is she should never have had the second hand done or even the first, which never got the expected relief.

Many of you have already had the unpleasant experience of having surgery and not gotten better. There are myriad reasons for not improving from carpal tunnel surgery. One of the common reasons people do not improve or their symptoms do not go away is incomplete release of the ligament. Another reason is there is more nerve damage than simple release will cure.

Sometimes the diagnosis is just plain incorrect. Medicine is an art as well as a science. Often patients complain of nerve symptoms and it is just assumed their carpal tunnel problem is the main issue. Very often, indeed, the median nerve is not the culprit and certainly not the median nerve at the wrist level. Remember, these nerves start at the neck and travel down the arm to the forearm, wrist, and hand. Many times when surgery is not successful, it is because the diagnosis is incomplete. When this is the case, patients will get no relief or, at best, incomplete relief with a distal surgery. It is essential we look further to see just where the actual pathology is.

The problem of "recurrent carpal tunnel" requires an upper extremity specialist. Once you have had surgery and incomplete or no relief is the result, a new workup should begin. Once a completely thorough evaluation is performed, there are very few patients for whom we cannot confirm a diagnosis and at least give reasonable relief from the pain of nerve symptoms.

We see many patients who have been through multiple programs and surgeries and still have gotten no relief. These are not people who are desirous of continuing to be symptomatic but rather patients who do not fit the paradigms of the system. The nature of nerve problems and specifically multilevel nerve problems makes these issues complex and quite difficult to diagnose let alone treat. If you find yourself in the unfortunate circumstance of being one of these patients, the best thing to do is to begin all over again. A new workup from step one if necessary should be performed to try and pin down the true etiology of your problem. This will require not only your doctor but also you as a patient attempting to understand the nature and origin of your symptomatology.

Thoracic Outlet
Syndrome

CHAPTER 10

You would not be reading this book if you were not aware there are patients diagnosed as having carpal tunnel and who do not get better with standard medical care and treatment. We often see patients who present with nerve symptoms that are not classically "carpal tunnel problems." They have symptoms that do not fit the usual diagnostic criteria.

"Denise" was thrown across the street when she was hit by a bus. She sustained notable injuries but the most substantial were to her head, neck, and upper extremities. She had significant problems after the accident and an inability to use her hand and arm well. She had pain and was unable to write. Denise was studying sign language to work with the handicapped and also worked as a legal secretary.

She was given multiple diagnoses but ultimately her pathology was pinned down by a good team including a neurologist who understood complex nerve problems. She has been able to minimize her symptoms with medication but has remained with the severe pain of underlying nerve problems. Although her arm will never be normal, she has at least been able to go forward with her life against all odds. We were able to confirm

Denise's diagnosis as a significant thoracic outlet injury with damage to the internal structure of her nerves.

Denise is a dramatic example of a patient who developed thoracic outlet problems secondary to a severe injury. Most thoracic outlet injuries are much more subtle in presentation and onset. Many are confused with other nerve problems and pain syndromes. Many people look for a major insult to result in thoracic outlet syndrome instead of an onset with injury on a more subtle basis.

Today, the medical community and the public are very much aware of carpal tunnel. Remember the old adage *a little knowledge is a dangerous thing*. Further confusion arises in that diagnoses today are given before the doctor even sees the patient. People are "labeled" by everyone from ancillary medical personnel to insurance claim adjusters and company statisticians. These people are armed with outdated manuals and diagnosis codes that explain in very little, if any, detail the nature of nerve problems. What we have failed to teach them is all upper extremity nerve problems are *not* carpal tunnel.

In his book *The Seven Habits of Highly Successful People*, Stephen Covey talks about paradigms. Paradigms are simply accepted norms in our way of viewing things. They form the basis for our perceptions of all other events. For example, we all accept the paradigm when we get up out of bed, our feet will plant firmly on the ground. This paradigm is based on our understanding of gravity and on our experience on a daily basis. From the time we could get up and stand, gravity held us to the earth. If gravity were eliminated, our basic concept of dealing with getting out of bed in the morning would change quite a bit. This is one of the adaptations men and women have made in space flight.

The paradigm today concerning nerve problems is many consider all nerve problems in the arm to be related to the carpal tunnel. When a patient presents with symptoms outside of the norm of a carpal tunnel problem, he or she falls outside of the paradigm or basic orientation of most people who see nerve problems. When this occurs, not only does confusion ensue but also misdiagnosis and disbelief.

To remedy this situation, the basic paradigm for dealing with patients with nerve problems must be changed. The medical community, patients, insurance adjusters, employers, and all others who make decisions concerning these problems must be educated. It must be understood nerve problems do exist but each is a separate and individual entity. When a patient has nerve complaints and either does not respond to carpal tunnel surgery or has symptoms out of the norm as described for "carpal tunnel syndrome," this may be not only appropriate but exactly predictable based on clinical findings.

The basic paradigm for dealing with nerve problems should be that abnormal sensations do occur with the associated symptoms of pain, numbness, tingling, and motor dysfunction. In some cases, this may be carpal tunnel; in others, there may be more significant involvement, such as patients with thoracic outlet syndrome. It then becomes much easier to accept and understand complaints that appear somewhat bizarre when viewed from the standard paradigm "all nerve problems are related to the carpal tunnel." Once we realize this is an incorrect basis for assumptions, the rest falls into place.

As you recall from chapter 5, nerves begin at the neck and travel as long structures or cables through the arm to the fingertips. Anywhere along this circuit, compromise can occur and result in altered function. Scarring, inflammation, or compression between the neck and shoulder at the thoracic outlet level can produce nerve symptoms. These patients have many complaints overlapping those associated with distal nerve compressions, such as carpal tunnel at the wrist, cubital tunnel at the elbow involving the ulnar nerve, or radial tunnel at the forearm with radial nerve symptoms. Each results in symptoms in a different nerve distribution. When this occurs at the level of the thoracic outlet, any or all of these symptoms may present.

"Francine" complained of many symptoms consistent with carpal tunnel. She had numbness and tingling in her hands and inability to work at repetitive activities. Her job as a postal worker was highly repetitive. She recognized early on her symptoms were not a classical carpal tunnel problem. We undertook a therapy and treatment program for Francine and discovered her major problem was at the thoracic outlet level due to carrying mail bags on that shoulder and repetitive reaching activities. With substantial modifications in her lifestyle and no surgery whatsoever, we were able to improve her symptoms. She has continued to work for the U.S. Postal Service, although in a modified capacity. Had Francine gone strictly with the generally accepted protocols in medicine today, she would no doubt have had carpal tunnel surgery and continued to be symptomatic. If she had tried to return to her regular pre-injury job, she would have had recurrent problems and become another statistic rather than an improved and functional member of society.

The thoracic outlet is a tunnel or passage for all the nerves that go into the arm after they leave the spinal cord at the neck. It is located just behind the collarbone between the neck and shoulder. If you walk your fingers over your collarbone toward your back and note a hollow just behind the collarbone, this is the supraclavicular fossa. If you press lightly there, you actually can palpate (feel) the upper trunk of the brachial plexus. If you walk your fingers under and in front of the collarbone, this would be the area of the middle and lower trunk of the brachial plexus. The nerves are covered by muscle but they generally are palpable and we use this diagnostically. (Mr. Spock, of course, used this to his advantage with the Vulcan nerve pinch, but this is not part of our recommended treatment!)

The nerves are covered in front by a muscle called the anterior scalene. Embryologically (from conception through de-

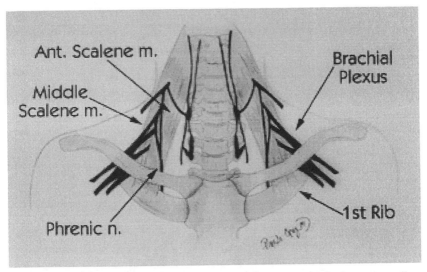

The thoracic outlet. Shown are the nerves of the brachial plexus traveling through the thoracic outlet bound in front by the anterior scalene muscle, beneath by the first rib and behind by the middle scalene muscle.

velopment of the nervous system), the nerves of the brachial plexus actually grow right through a muscle mass and this mass divides becoming the anterior, middle, and posterior scalene muscles. Suffice it to say, these muscles surround the nerves of the brachial plexus and, as do many nerves in the body, glide and move between the layers of these muscle groups. Along with nerves of the brachial plexus travels the subclavian artery through the same thoracic outlet (tunnel) area. This artery supplies blood to the arm. The thoracic outlet is bound below by the first rib, posteriorly (in the back) by the middle scalene, and anteriorly (in front) by the anterior scalene muscle. This essentially forms a triangle through which the nerve structures travel (see diagram).

Injury to the nerves of the brachial plexus may occur in a number of different ways. Whiplash-type injuries, as people sustain in car accidents, with flexion (looking down), extension (looking up), or side-bending injuries of the neck may result in tearing of the scalene muscle proper and/or yanking or ripping

131

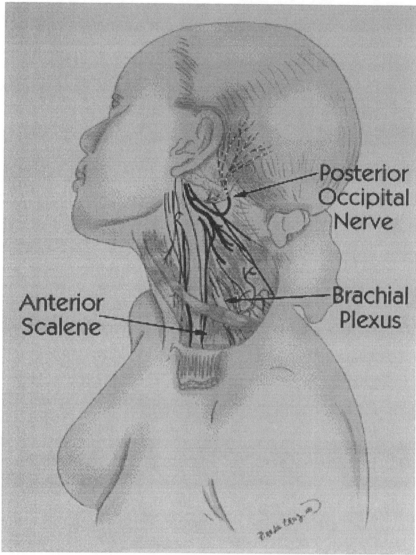

The anterior scalene muscle is seen here covering the nerves of the brachial plexus. Seen also are the posterior occipital branches to the head which are often symptomatic causing headaches.

of the normal fine cobweb scar tissue which holds the nerves of the brachial plexus in place. This scar tissue in its normal state is called fascia and holds the nerves in place so they do not clang around in the chest cavity. When this tissue about the nerves is torn or the muscle itself around the nerves is injured, inflammation ensues and a thicker adherent tissue may form binding down the nerves of the plexus, resulting in symptoms such as pain, discomfort, and disability.

"Manny" originally came to me when he injured his shoulder. We performed surgery to stabilize his shoulder for chronic dislocations. He did well with this and was able to pursue various jobs and activities. Unfortunately, Manny is one of those people who always walks around with a black cloud over his head. He calls it his "Charlie Brown syndrome."

He sustained his latest injury while he was working on some scaffolding and slipped and fell. He tried to catch himself with his already compromised arm. He ended up with his full weight on this arm in a completely extended (abducted) position over his head. This caused a yanking and tractioning injury to the brachial plexus. No one believed his complaints of numbness and pain or even considered the diagnosis of a brachial plexus problem. We were ultimately able to convince everyone he had sustained a significant injury and his nerve studies were markedly positive, indicating severe injury to the nerves of his thoracic outlet.

Manny did nicely with therapy and conservative care. Although his arm remained numb for many months, he did come around and is now back to full function and working. He is also now a father and his positive attitude has paid off in more than one way. Manny also has the great benefit of a wonderful and supportive wife. There is no doubt they, as a team, are responsible for his continued ability to bounce back from his multiple significant injuries.

Brachial plexus problems may occur in a much more subtle way with repetitive minor traumas such as repeatedly reaching (as scanning in a grocery store), the use of jackhammers, and hammering. Yanking or pulling injuries on the arm may also result in tearing of these tissues. Direct blows to the shoulder or plexus area can cause the same type injuries as well.

"Anna" was standing around minding her own business when she was injured. She was leaning against a light post in a wet area. A short in the system caused her to be the conductor of electricity and she sustained a direct electrical injury to her brachial plexus. This resulted in an acute spasm and tearing of the scalene muscle and injury to the muscles surrounding and also the nerves of the brachial plexus. The result was significant scarring and damage to these nerves.

Anna developed continued and progressive symptomatology and became severely uncomfortable. She was significantly limited in her ability to perform any activities that required reaching, pulling, pushing, or any regular use of the arm. She had severe problems with headaches, pain, and discomfort. We placed her in a therapy program, but she did not get complete relief. She subsequently underwent distal arm surgery at her carpal canal and at her ulnar nerve at the elbow to try and give her some relief. Although she got some temporary partial relief, we were not able to give her any good relief at the plexus level or relief from her severe symptoms, which continued to progress.

Anna reached a point where she felt her situation unlivable, and although the surgery does carry with it a high risk, she felt she would rather risk the possible consequences of the surgery at the brachial plexus level than live with her symptoms. We then had the unfortunate circumstance of having to convince her insurance carrier surgery was the proper thing to do. Because of the significant controversies surrounding this complex and highly intricate surgery, as well as the lack of understanding personally on her insurance adjuster's part, we spent almost six months obtaining approval for her surgery. Anna became quite depressed at her situation and her inability to get relief from her continued pain.

Anna is a strong-willed and bold lady and in spite of all the road blocks put in front of her, she knew in her heart this was the proper way for her to go. She was able to communicate to me the strength of her convictions, and although it required an extensive amount of pressure on our part, we finally were able to obtain approval for her to have surgery.

During surgery, we not only documented the suspected damage but we were able to rectify it. She had almost immediate relief from her severe pain as soon as the nerves were freed. She went back to work two weeks after her surgery, which is an extraordinarily rapid recovery. She continues to do well and has taught me and my patients just what attitude and determination can bring in life.

It is important to remember injury or pathology about the nerves of the brachial plexus can reproduce any of the symptoms we may classically see from compression or scarring about any of the nerves in the arm. The site of conduction delay causing "symptoms" is simply interpreted at the cerebral cortex (brain) level, and it is often impossible for patient and physician to tell exactly where the nerve entrapment has occurred. It is up to the medical community to define clinically exactly where the "short," or pathology, is in the circuit.

A further complicating factor is the sympathetic nerves enter the arm through the nerve of Kuhns at the lower trunk of the brachial plexus. This results in many patients with thoracic outlet or brachial plexus problems exhibiting other symptoms and signs that do not fit classical nerve distributions and described clinical pictures. They show problems such as color changes in the hand, swelling, variations in temperature of the hand and arm, and the like. They are often confused with reflex sympathetic dystrophy patients or, worse, as overreactive or pain-syndrome patients and treated as the same.

The key to diagnosing and treating thoracic outlet or brachial plexus problems is simply listening to the patient and the story of their injury. If allowed to describe the nature of their complaints, patients generally within five minutes clearly define a thoracic outlet or brachial plexus problem. Those with thoracic outlet problems regularly complain of symptoms with overhead activities, reaching, pulling, pushing, and lifting. They often describe activities such as combing or blow drying their hair as being impossible and causing their arms to go numb. Many have actually arranged their homes in different ways so dishes are on lower shelves. Any activities that involve reaching overhead are simply out of the question. These patients have significant fatiguability in their arms. They often have overlapping symptoms of night pain and discomfort but when we speak further, they usually relate awaking with numbness and their arms in an overhead position or they were sleeping on the involved side. Driving is often problematic for these patients, and this again is consistent with the posturing of the arms and neck.

"Vinny" had severe pain and discomfort because of a serious brachial plexus problem but was simply not the kind of man who gave in to pain. Getting to know Vinny over the course of time, I became aware of the fact he had been a paratrooper and in charge of a unit during the Vietnam war. He had been responsible for the lives of many men and saw them through multiple life-and-death situations. In fact, when it came time to do Vinny's thoracic outlet surgery, we discussed the possible complications of the operation; he stated to me very matter-of-factly, "I faced death many times before and this is an easy choice. I can't live with my pain any longer so the decision is obvious."

Vinny went on to do well post-operatively and obtained relief from his surgery. Somehow, however, we were never quite able to bring him to complete relief. On further discussions with Vinny, I came to realize he was born and raised in Kentucky. He had been displaced, due to work and other issues, to the

East Coast. After much soul-searching, we both decided part of his healing process had to be to return to his home. Although we had freed his nerves and given them the chance to heal, we had not freed his mind to heal appropriately. I last heard from Vinny about six months ago. The return home did him a world of good and helped him bridge the last gap in complete healing. This was a decision he and I came to realize only after extensive discussions. Had I not been afforded the privilege of knowing him as a person as well as a patient, I doubt we would have ever been able to bring Vinny that last mile to obtain better relief for him from the pain in his body.

When I listen further to patients with thoracic outlet problems, they will often give a history of progressive problems. Their symptoms evolve over the course of time and are the result of cumulative trauma problems or repetitive motion disorders. Patients often relate their hands or wrists initially bothered them, and they were given splints by a well-meaning friend or physician. They continued to perform repetitive activities or jobs and instead of using the wrist motions, which were taken away by the splint, began using their elbows repetitively. The elbows over the course of time became uncomfortable, and these patients often develop problems at the radial tunnel or lateral epicondyle about the extensor origin, such as tennis elbow. They may develop problems on the inner medial side of the arm along the lines of ulnar nerve involvement or cubital tunnel. Then they attempt not to move their elbows on a regular basis and start overusing the shoulder. There is much more reaching, and gross whole arm motions substitute for finer dexterous lower arm use. Activities once done easily are performed in awkward or bizarre postures to compensate for the pain. At this point, the nerves are being yanked or pulled at the level of the brachial plexus and the problem becomes unlivable. Progressive inflammation, swelling, and scarring about these nerves occurs and ultimately they develop full-blown thoracic outlet syndrome.

"Melanie" spent 20 years working as a checker for a large food chain and openly brags she was "the best checker they ever had." She was always in the fastest line and won awards on multiple occasions for being the fastest and most successful cashier. She is also a very astute and bright lady. She had worked with the union in her organization and helped many people with "carpal tunnel problems" find their way off the lines. She came to realize very early on in her career as a union person that many of these people had surgery and did not get better.

Melanie began to notice her hands were becoming problematic. The numbness progressed and reached the point where she wasn't able to feel the grain on the money as it passed through her fingers. This, she related, is essential to detect counterfeit bills. She came to see me with one of the worst cases of multiple level nerve scarring I've ever encountered. Melanie is a true example of a cumulative trauma problem. She initially had problems with her hands and wrists and modified her checking and working style. She used splints and repeatedly abused her elbows on an overuse basis to continue her rapid pace. When her elbows hurt, she just reached further and got her neck and shoulders involved, thereby completing the three levels of nerve disease.

Melanie's EMGs are markedly positive. She has already had surgery at the carpal tunnel level. Although Melanie has gotten some relief with these surgeries, as expected, she remains with symptoms. She has modified her life substantially. She is now a shop steward and has not gone back to the activities that caused her problems. Melanie still has pain on a daily basis although using biofeedback relaxation techniques and continuing with a wonderfully positive mental attitude, Melanie has been able to live her life, raise her children, care for her husband, and maintain an extraordinarily upbeat personality.

She always has a smile and although she lives with pain, Melanie feels she is better doing this than risking further surgery. Ultimately, Melanie may come to thoracic outlet surgery. However, she may be one of those people whose lifestyle modification and extraordinary will afford her enough relief to avoid surgical intervention at the brachial plexus level.

If we catch this sequence of events early on, we not only avoid the development of a full-blown thoracic outlet problem but can actually reverse the symptomatology. Indeed this is the key to treating any of the cumulative trauma problems or multi-level neuropathies. When the patients are taken out of the offending environment and taught how to modify their lifestyles and activities, they are very often able to obtain relief from the symptoms.

What we need to remember is nerves have a wonderful innate capacity to heal themselves. Given the proper environment and treatment, many nerve problems will calm down and actually reverse their damage. It is only when the inflammation and swelling about these nerves reach the point of significant scarring and compression, and these nerves are not free to glide or move normally in the tissues, these nerve problems become fixed or permanent and require surgical intervention. It is important to remember once we reach a point of requiring surgical intervention, we lose the game. This does not mean we lose the whole series but indeed this becomes a more significant situation and the expectations for recovery and return to full function become much less predictable. Understanding this, we realize why lifestyle modification needs to be the first and foremost option in treatment. Even when we perform surgery, it is not advisable for most to return to the activities that caused the nerve problem in the first place.

A Brief History

There are many today who look at thoracic outlet problems as a new diagnosis. In fact, the diagnosis and treatment of thoracic outlet problems dates back to the late 1800s. The first thoracic outlet surgery was performed in the 1890s. Over the ensuing 100 years, many people have undergone thoracic outlet surgery and improved. Some have not done so well.

In the early 1900s, Dr. A.W. Adson did a good deal of work with thoracic outlet problems and some confusion existed as to the underlying pathology. He believed this was mainly a vascular problem in that he used a decrease in the amplitude of the pulse when bringing the arm out and away from the body as a confirmation of his diagnosis. He recommended surgical treatment only when a loss of pulse could be documented. This misconception is still followed by some today.

Dr. David Roos popularized first-rib resection in the mid-1900s based on decompressing the artery and the brachial plexus from below in the axilla or arm pit. He helped bring back the understanding that the main problem is one of nerve entrapment and is not vascular in most cases. This was a great breakthrough, and indeed Dr. Roos is responsible for helping many people with thoracic outlet problems. The first-rib resection, however, is a procedure that carries substantial possible complications including bleeding problems, pneumothorax (dropping or collapse of the lung), and partial or complete paralysis if nerve structures are pulled or yanked too aggressively from below. In some hands, this remains a good procedure and helpful for thoracic outlet problems, especially in lower trunk involvement.

In the late 1970s, Dr. James Hunter along with Dr. Stephan Whitenack and Dr. Scott Jaeger defined a different approach to the thoracic outlet. They pursued the premise this was basically a nerve entrapment problem and the scarring about these nerves was a significant aspect of the pathology. They believed simply decompressing (opening up) the outlet from below was not adequate. It was recommended that looking at the nerves proper and freeing the scar tissue was the best way to go. In fact, this brought us almost full circle back to the late 1800s when thoracic outlet syndrome was recognized as a nerve problem. Dr. Hunter and his associates undertook a supraclavicular approach and recommended complete removal of the anterior scalene muscle, which is the compression force over the nerves. Once the nerves are exposed, freeing them by performing a neurolysis (removing the scar around them) is then performed.

This procedure is safer with fewer complications affording predictable relief to many of these patients. The complication rate for the supraclavicular approach is less because the nerves and vessels are directly visualized. While this is generally sufficient, some patients may require this procedure along with first rib resection. We have found using the supraclavicular approach, approximately 80 percent of patients are able to get relief from their symptoms. Although this is a safer procedure, it is still an operation that should be undertaken only in extreme circumstances; possible complications of any thoracic outlet surgery are significant, including paralysis, bleeding problems, pneumothorax, and even death.

I came to know "Perry" a few years ago. An inmate at a local prison, he had developed chronic renal failure and could not afford the dialysis treatments he required. I was asked to see him because he had severe pain in his hand which was radiating up his arm. The initial consultation instructions from the patient were to arrange to "cut off his arm." Of course, I felt this was a bit drastic.

Communication was somewhat difficult since Perry was Greek, and my only way of communicating with him was through one of the nurses in the hospital who happened to speak the language fluently. I tried to tell him there were other options. He insisted the only way to relieve the pain was to take the entire arm off. In fact, his main disease was in the tip of one of his fingers and a second whole finger in the hand. We compromised, and because these fingers were essentially gangrenous (with no blood to them at all), we began with the fingers. I told him we would work our way up the arm if necessary.

Perry had an underlying nerve problem and a significant pain issue. Although he wasn't the most cooperative patient, we actually got his fingers to heal and did rid him of his pain.

This was no doubt a difficult relationship to form; communication being only one of multiple issues with Perry. I learned from him, however, that referred pain (which travels along nerves to different areas) is not generally straight forward. Many times, what appears to be a limb-threatening problem is simply a matter of pinpointing where the majority of the pain is coming from and treating it. Perry certainly was better off losing a finger or two than the entire extremity.

Perry's desire to lose a limb rather than feel the pain is not unusual. Physicians often joke about the "requirements" for patients to have thoracic outlet surgery. I have heard it described by more than one person that patients should not consider having thoracic outlet surgery until they reach a point where the pain is so bad they want you to cut off their arm. This obviously indicates the significant nature of the pain with the thoracic outlet problems and descriptively indicates the point patients need to reach before considering this type of risky surgery.

What has become apparent to me is the medical community has become stagnant in its thinking concerning nerve problems since the 1950s when Dr. Phalen popularized carpal tunnel as an entity. Doctors and patients became focused on nerve problems as being related to the carpal tunnel. Somehow since that time, we segmented our thinking through specialization. Neurosurgeons concentrated on disc problems at the neck level and hand surgeons focused on the carpal tunnel at the wrist. Further confounding the issue were vascular surgeons performing the rib resections for thoracic outlet problems. This led to a fragmentation of the thought processes, each group forgetting about the other end of the arm. It became similar to the blind men describing the elephant. The person at the level of the trunk described an elephant as being like a snake. The one at his body described it as being like a truck and the man at the tail as a feathered ostrich. Without treating the whole patient and looking at the entire picture, we could not clearly and easily recognize, diagnose, and treat nerve problems.

Dr. Hunter and his colleagues took this work further, and I was privileged to have trained with him. He helped us to see the whole picture once again and more clearly.

What we realize now is we *must* evaluate patients from their fingertips all the way to the neck. There are patients who have disc problems and do require spine surgery. There are also patients who simply have carpal tunnel problems and require treatment solely at that level. Unfortunately, many patients fall in the middle, and these are the patients who often fall through the cracks of today's medical system. Too often patients with thoracic outlet problems go undiagnosed. I am at times amazed patients come to me after years of treatment when no one has ever evaluated or examined them for any problems higher than the wrist. This is not to say the physicians treating them were bad doctors, but rather these patients were treated by people who, due to either the overwhelming time constraints in medical practice or the lack of specific training, simply missed the diagnosis.

"Kevin" is a 25-year-old warehouse manager. He developed severe problems with numbness and cramping in his hands as well as a burning sensation that was awakening him at night. When he attempted increased work at his job, he had substantially more symptomatology.

Kevin was a highly motivated young man and did not only a good deal of manual work in the warehouse but also landscaping work on the side for the owner of the company. He was advancing well in the company but unfortunately at the cost of his hands and arms. His nerve study showed severe positivity, and there was no doubt he was headed toward a substantial multi-level nerve problem if he didn't change his course.

Kevin and I had extensive discussions as to options for his arms. He and I both agreed avoiding operative intervention would be best. We discussed ways to try and modify his lifestyle and yet maintain his good standing with his boss. Kevin explained the situation to his employer. He related he very much enjoyed his job as well as their relationship and wished to do anything he could to help his boss and move his company forward. The boss, to his credit, recognized his talent and eagerness to achieve. I think he also recognized his good common sense. Kevin was actually promoted to a higher managerial job and advanced his status in the company. He was using night splints and stopped doing the landscaping. He was able to both achieve an advanced position in his job and also avoid surgery. Kevin did very well using his brains rather than his brawn and did not sacrifice his body for advancement.

I often tell patients in a half-joking manner that there are only three things people are willing to pay you for in this world. The first is to beat up your body and abuse it. People are paid well to wear out their bodies rapidly. The second is for their brains, common sense, and the ideas they may come up with. The third thing people are willing to pay for is educational status and experience. Unfortunately, many people from professional athletes to pill packers fall into the first category. Many times, this pays well in the short term but in the long run results in severe long-term problems as we've described.

Most patients with thoracic outlet problems are able to resolve their symptoms on a conservative basis. Once the diagnosis is made, a well-oriented treatment program aimed at nerve gliding and exercises to decrease the amount of compression and stretch the scar tissue about these nerves often results in good relief of pain and symptoms.

"James" was a large truck mechanic and worked aggressively with his arms for many years. Unfortunately, the years took their toll, and James developed severe problems in both right and left arms with not only distal nerve involvement but also thoracic outlet syndrome bilaterally. He underwent extensive treatment with respect to his pain and nerve disease and had surgeries on his hands and wrists, elbows, and the thoracic outlet. Although we have been able to give James some relief from the severe pain he had, his arms are still not normal.

James, however, is a wonderful example of a person who has changed his entire attitude and concept about life. He is a family man and I say this is in the true sense. He has a very supportive wife who has a wonderful sense of humor. The shift James and his wife have made is in raising their boys. He has become much more involved as a mainstay of the family at home and she has continued her radiology career. James is an individual who is able to maintain his identity and self-worth through his family. He has accepted the fact he will never return to his mechanic job. He plans to further his education to pursue alternative careers. In the meantime, he has accepted a temporary change in his status making this beneficial not only to himself but also to his family. He is an inspiration to me and many of my patients and I applaud him and his ability to adapt. James has taken a situation that would have destroyed many people and made it a positive issue for all those who are important to him.

Our extensive program is aimed at lifestyle modification as well as biofeedback relaxation techniques, therapy modalities, and exercises aimed at freeing these nerves proper. It has been our experience most patients do not require thoracic outlet surgery and only 5 to 10 percent of patients who come to us with a diagnosis of thoracic outlet problems require surgical intervention at that level.

Most thoracic outlet problems are based on multiple levels of nerve involvement. Safer, less risky surgeries when done appropriately and in the appropriate order are often successful in relieving symptoms enough to either allow the nerves at the thoracic outlet level to heal or at least decrease the intensity of symptoms. It has been our experience, clinically, that 50 percent of patients who have adequate freeing of the median nerve at the wrist level get this expected relief. Another 70 percent of patients who have decompression of the ulnar nerve at the elbow when involved get good relief of their proximal thoracic outlet symptoms. What must be remembered here is these patients get relief from their symptoms but often are not returned to the type of activities that caused their problems in the first place. They understand the nature of their problem and have utilized therapy and lifestyle modifications aimed at helping to calm these nerves from the neck and brachial plexus level all the way down to the hand and wrist. The therapy program is as important, if not more, than the surgeries themselves. The patient must understand the nature of multi-level nerve involvement and exactly how this can be taken care of.

Thoracic outlet syndrome, as an entity, does exist and has so for many years. The very nature of this problem helps explain many of the signs and symptoms present in patients who do not follow the classic patterns of the commonly seen lower arm nerve compression problems.

Pain Syndromes and Reflex Sympathetic Dystrophy

CHAPTER 11

"Man is sometimes extraordinarily, passionately, in love with suffering."

—Dostoevsky

It is hoped by this point you have a fairly good understanding of nerve problems and are aware most problems with respect to nerve issues have an underlying, identifiable, physiologic basis. There are, however, patients who simply do not fit any of the normal physiologic patterns and, after thorough workups, do not have an identifiable cause for their pain, discomfort, and disease. These are patients with true pain syndromes and, at times, reflex sympathetic dystrophy (RSD).

"Valerie" described the cyclical pattern of pain problems very well. She had been living with her symptoms for a number of years and noted significant progression of her pain. She described her problem as one of not being able to function well on a long-term basis. She told me she felt her life was basically going nowhere.

She was unable to sleep at night and was awakened every few hours. She had fallen into a pattern of watching television until late at night. When she finally fell asleep, she awoke every few hours with pain that continued throughout the night. By the morning, she had significantly increased pain as well as irritability. She has continued to try and work at her regular job. Getting showered and dressed took her an extraordinarily long time. When she got to work, Valerie was exhausted and unable to perform her regular duties. When she got home, she was barely able to make herself a meal. Then the night cycle began all over again.

Valerie wept as she described her frustration at not being able to enjoy anything in life. She described her life as just "walking through day to day with no enjoyment." This appeared to be what was dragging her down faster than anything else. She got occasional relief with medications but realized the answer was to break the pattern.

Many of the symptoms of these pain syndromes and RSD overlap those of nerve compression problems. Specifically, patients with RSD often present with numbness, tingling, pain, and discomfort as well as swelling and color changes in the hands. The differential is often hard to make. The nerve of Kuhns carries sympathetic innervation to the upper extremity through the thoracic outlet. This makes thoracic outlet syndrome an even more challenging diagnostic dilemma. Since many of the symptoms of RSD overlap those of thoracic outlet and nerve compression problems, we again see the need for a complete workup prior to diagnosing someone as having RSD or a pain syndrome.

It is imperative to remember there are many patients with sympathetic reactivity in their arms who do not have RSD or pain syndromes. A physiologic and neurologic basis should always be ruled out before labeling patients as RSD or sending them off to a pain program. All too often I see patients who have been misdiagnosed and labeled as RSD or pain syndrome patients. Many have been through pain programs and spent years waiting for their "RSD to resolve." They found out, unfortunately quite late, they actually had underlying physiologic nerve problems that had gone undiagnosed. Once these patients with true disease were placed in pain programs, they entered what I call the "pain program cycle." They became casualties of the medical system.

Another of my patients had a severe brachial plexus problem. She was on low doses of elavil, which is a medication originally marketed for depression but helps with sleep and decreases the intensity of nerve pain. She utilized biofeedback/pain management techniques and medications just to survive. She described the past year as being "like a nightmare I can't wake up from." She related, "I dance with the pain so it won't get the best of me."

It never ceases to amaze me just how many patients have never had a thorough evaluation prior to being placed in pain programs. I find, very often, after reviewing copious records, no one has even performed an exam on these patients at the neck, thoracic-outlet, or upper-arm level. Very often the only examinations performed are at the hand and wrist and the only thing ruled in or out is the presence of a carpal tunnel problem. No evaluation for ulnar or radial nerve problems at the elbow, thoracic outlet, or cervical disc problems has been made prior to placing these patients in pain programs and writing them off. It is unfortunate, but once these people are placed in the pain program cycle, there is little hope of getting them back to becoming functional family members or members of the working society because they are being treated from the wrong approach.

It is not uncommon for patients to break down and cry when I tell them there is an underlying nerve problem and they are not crazy. The final straw is when I tell them there is actually something that can be done to help them. These are generally frustrated patients who have lost their faith and trust in the medical system and physicians. These people have sim-

149

ply fallen through the cracks of the medical system and are often labeled as malingers, abusers, crazy, or worse.

"Lorena" is a social worker who sustained significant injury to her right hand, wrist, and arm while trying to break up a fight among clients. She had a severe wrist injury as well as progressive nerve problems in her arm. Her arm became totally dysfunctional. She was told by the surgeon who operated on her there was absolutely nothing wrong with her hand anymore. She was informed it was impossible for her to ever have recurrence of disease or problems and since her carpal tunnel was "fixed," all the rest of her pain was in her head.

Unfortunately, Lorena was a trusting person and she took this to heart. She was under the impression nothing further could be done for her arm and attempted to push through and abuse her arm even though there was actually real physiologic disease still present. When I met Lorena, she was unable to move her wrist at all and kept it bent all the way down in a flexed position. She had poor hand function, significant nerve symptoms, and pain.

After three surgeries, hundreds of hours of therapy, and an excellent support system at home, Lorena has made quite a bit of progress. I think she has taught me as much about healing and motivation techniques as we've taught her. Once we were able to move forward, having Lorena understand the relationship of herself to her pain, she was able to give herself relief.

The Differential Diagnosis of Reflex Sympathetic Dystrophy

There are many patients who indeed do have reflex sympathetic dystrophy. RSD is a problem hallmarked by pain, swelling, and reactive changes in the arms. The classic description of this is pain out of proportion to the nature and/or degree of the injury.

150

In further defining reflex sympathetic dystrophy, it is helpful to understand what I term *sympathetic* reactivity, a component of the reflex *sympathetic* dystrophy issue. You may recall when you were in grade school your teacher described the "fight or flight" mechanism. Picture a scenario where you are walking down a dark street in a not-so-good neighborhood at about 1:00 A.M. You are lost and the area is poorly lit. As you pass by an alleyway someone jumps out in front of you. Your body prepares for either "fight" or "flight." Essentially your heart begins to beat faster and your blood vessels dilate to increase the circulation to your arm and leg muscles. The nerves at the tips of your fingers and your arms actually became heightened in sensitivity for better tactile response. Your eyes become wide open with your pupils dilated to take in any activity and action that might occur. You may even begin to sweat at this point, and there is a significant surge in intensity of all of your senses. This is your sympathetic nervous system in action.

In patients with sympathetic reactivity or RSD, this sympathetic activity continues unbridled. There is no control over this and basically there is a short-circuit in the system. Instead of calming down once the apparent danger and/or injury has left, this system continues to re-activate itself and produce the responses noted above. This is hallmarked by the increased sensitivity and irritability of the nerves, which account for the pain. The swelling, color changes and increased reactivity to touch all are consistent with this as well. I have often described patients as having sympathetic reactivity rather than full-blown RSD in that there are many gradations of sympathetic reactivity. Everyone with these reactive changes in the arms does not have a full-blown reflex sympathetic dystrophy and is not doomed to the fate we see in older textbooks that label this problem as causalgia, shoulder/hand syndrome, Sudek's atrophy, and the like.

Early in my career, I had a most frightening experience with reflex sympathetic dystrophy. A good friend who was also the wife of one of the prominent physicians in the hospital where I work sustained a small fracture in her hand. When I saw her in the office, "Janice" said her hand was okay and whatever I thought we should do was fine with her. I spoke with her husband who informed me in no uncertain terms he wanted her treated exactly as I would any other patient. You see, in the medical community, we often try to get around formal treatments and take shortcuts we feel would be "easier on those we know." This is an unfortunate mistake and very often the care ends up altered to the point where it is harmful.

I took her husband's advice and recommended a pinning of the fracture to stabilize it. This would allow the earliest motion and also the least time in a cast or immobilization. Unfortunately, because of her fracture, Janice developed a full-blown reflex sympathetic dystrophy. She had severe pain, swelling, color changes, and reactivity in the hand and arm.

As you can well imagine, it being early in my career, I was not pleased. I saw a friend in pain and my future in the hospital disappearing before my eyes.

Luckily for me, Janice is an extraordinarily strong-willed lady and was also willing to travel a great distance to obtain appropriate therapy not readily available in our community. After six months of hard work and aggressive physical therapy as well as emotional support (the latter for both of us), Janice obtained full function of her hand and resolution of her sympathetic dystrophy (pain).

We have at times diagnosed patients as having "pain syndromes" because we really do not have a diagnosis for them. There are patients who simply do not fall into any of the categories we have available in the way of diagnoses. This is not to say these patients do not have pain, but rather they have pain of a nature and basis for which we have no discernable cause.

These may be patients who have forms of RSD or nerve dysfunction we are simply not able to diagnose. If you are diagnosed as a pain patient, this does not mean you are crazy. It simply means the underlying basis for your pain is out of the scope of our current medical understanding. This does not mean you should give up on yourself, but rather you should take advantage of the available alternative treatments and programs to level out your pain.

"Tom," a former bus driver, is one such example. He sustained severe injury when the hydraulic mechanism that opens bus doors malfunctioned and literally picked him up off the ground yanking his right arm up and crushing him between his bus and another next to it. Although it was not amputated, he sustained significant crushing injury to the arm as well as a yanking or tractioning injury to the nerves of his brachial plexus.

Tom was initially treated conservatively but had progressive problems with the arm. He related a severe burning sensation, pain, and numbness. There were color changes in the arm and increased sweating and swelling. At night he was awakened from sleep with numbness and tingling in his arm, and it became severely and progressively more painful. He reached a point where he was unable to hold even a coffee cup and was dropping things. He had progressive symptoms in the way of pain, discomfort, and complete disability in the hand and arm.

When I first met Tom, his posture was such that he held his head off to the right trying to cradle it with his right shoulder, which was held up next to his ear. He maintained his right hand in a clenched fist and supported his arm in his lap by holding it close to his body. He had severe shaking and tremoring in the arm when he attempted to use it or move it away from his body. He was unable to make a full fist or bring his arm out very well away from his body without severe pain and discomfort.

153

To make matters worse, approximately three months after his initial injury, he broke his ankle and had to use crutches. This significantly progressed the pain and discomfort he had in his arm.

We maintained Tom in a therapy program and his nerve studies showed significant evidence of median nerve involvement at the wrist and also a traction injury with scarring about the nerves of his brachial plexus proper. He remained with severe symptoms in the arm and a low-level reflex sympathetic dystrophy as well, although he did not have a classic full-blown RSD picture.

Eventually, we performed surgery on Tom's arm for full mobilization of the median and ulnar nerve at the right hand and wrist at the level of the carpal tunnel. He got some relief with respect to his lower hand and arm pain but not with his upper arm and plexus. This was an expected possibility we had discussed prior to surgery and Tom remained with the same severe pain and discomfort he had pre-operatively.

Tom is unfortunately one of those people who has severe damage to the nerves of his arm and brachial plexus. He is not a candidate for further surgery in that he has such poor motion. He is truly a patient with a pain syndrome, and although we know he has internal structural damage to his nerves, we do not at this time have a cure for this problem. Although he is an exception rather than the rule, there are indeed patients like Tom who have pain for which we have no present cure. We have continued to encourage Tom not to lose hope and if he can one day reach a point where he is able to increase the motion in his arm and becomes a candidate for surgery, there may be some possibility of relief.

Patients with pain syndromes present a challenge, and this is exactly what pain programs were set up for. Treatments such as alternative medicines, nerve blocks, biofeedback, hypnosis, and the like are available. Most pain eventually levels

154

and burns out, especially if there is no physiologic basis for it. In these cases, it is indeed appropriate to continue with a pain program.

I often tell my patients in a somewhat joking manner it is my job to simply keep them sane long enough to allow their bodies to heal. In essence, in many cases, this is the reality of the situation. Pain syndromes as well as RSD are classic examples of issues that ultimately burn themselves out but often leave significant physical as well as emotional scars on patients. One hopes most of these scars are not inflicted by physicians in the name of healing.

Dr. Robert Schwartzman is a world authority on reflex sympathetic dystrophy. He has done an extensive amount of work concerning the treatment of RSD, and has helped us to understand there is a broad spectrum of disease that incorporates reflex sympathetic dystrophy. Previous thinking limited this to a single syndrome with only severe consequences, but we have learned through Dr. Schwartzman's work there is a wide variety of presentation of RSD. Many patients exhibit only some of the classic symptoms or lower levels of pain. These patients often fall into the category of those who can be helped and whose disease will go away or improve if it is recognized and treated. Dr. Schwartzman has helped us to understand many of these patients diagnosed as RSD have true nerve involvement, especially of the nerves of the thoracic outlet. He has pointed out the Kuhns nerve enters the upper extremity through the brachial plexus. This carries the sympathetic (reflex *sympathetic* dystrophy) fibers to the arm explaining why the clinical pictures of RSD and TOS patients are often so similar. He has been a great help in understanding these diseases from both a patient's and a physician's point of view.

Reflex sympathetic dystrophy is generally recognized as being broken down into three stages:

Stage I covers the time of injury to approximately six months afterward. This stage is marked by severe pain and re-activity. There is generally burning pain often described as out of proportion to the injury sustained. These patients present with color changes in the hand and arm and pain with any motion. The pain often radiates up and down the involved extremity. There is significant "autonomic instability" involving sweating and color changes as well as spasms in the hand and arm.

This is a critical stage because if the problem is recognized very early on and treatment is undertaken, the symptoms and problem can often be controlled. Patients may recover with minimal if any residual problems if treated aggressively. The key to treatment of stage I is early therapy and appropriate medications in the way of analgesics, anti-inflammatories, and at times oral corticosteroids and stellate ganglion nerve blocks when appropriate. Even in the best of circumstances and with early care, with severe RSD, it may not be possible to obtain a complete cure.

Stage II RSD encompasses many of the manifestations seen in stage I. The pattern of the pain and symptoms may often spread. This is the stage where we see such things as altered hair growth patterns and dystrophic changes in the hand, nails, and skin. The severe acute pain is not always there but the swelling and reactivity is often still present. Often these patients have significant evidence of what is termed "brawny edema" with marked stiffness in the joints of the fingers and hand. There is a shiny consistency to the skin and pain and discomfort with any attempt at motion.

Stage III RSD is essentially the end stage. The severe pain is generally decreased although these patients may continue to have significant pain and discomfort. This stage may go on for years or never entirely resolve. Even when therapy has been performed and the patient has gotten appropriate treatment, he or she may be left with significant residua in the way of stiffness, contractures, and reactive changes in the arm. There is usually some thickening of the subcutaneous tissues about the joints proper. Radiographic (X-ray) changes are usually seen between stages II and III with decreased mineralization in the bones. It is at this stage patients need to pursue aggressive attempts at lifestyle changes and move back toward normal life activities.

If you or someone you know carries a diagnosis of RSD or a "pain syndrome" and has been through a thorough and appropriate program for treating this but still has symptoms, it may be worthwhile to consider starting all over. Many times it is helpful to undergo a full physiologic as well as diagnostic evaluation once again to rule out any underlying pathology rather than to continue to work within the limitations of a diagnosis that may be only partially correct. Too often we see patients who have been treated on a course and once chartered never is corrected for shifts in wind or current. The people treating them simply follow that same program regardless of progress. After a period of time, it sometimes becomes apparent that course is leading nowhere.

As I have stated previously, the most important issue in the recovery of any patient is maintaining his or her desire to do just that—recover. As long as there is a desire to find the underlying cause of the problem and you continue to search for this, you will likely find a way to get better and be rid of your pain.

Remember reflex sympathetic dystrophy as well as pain syndromes with no underlying physiologic basis are extraordinarily rare. Most patients have underlying physiologic problems that can be treated. All that is necessary is to simply identify these and begin appropriate treatment.

Biofeedback, Hypnosis, and Magic

CHAPTER 12

*"If one advances confidently
in the direction of his dreams,
and endeavors to live the life
which he has imagined,
he will meet with success
unexpected in common hours."*

—Henry David Thoreau

Versatility, a broad knowledge base, and open-mindedness are the hallmark of the exceptional physician. To conceive a healer as having only a few medications in his or her repertoire and using them for any and all disorders may sound farfetched, but in this era of specialized training, physicians have become more and more channeled into their approach and view of patients and disease. I've often heard it said if the only tool you have at hand is a hammer, most things begin to look more and more like nails.

In an interview with Stephen Covey, Anthony Robbins spoke about paradigms and how they shape our belief processes and reactions to various situations. He relates a story about Mikhael Gorbachev. Robbins had asked Gorbachev how he had managed to change the relationship between Russia and the United States from antagonistic to its present state. He wondered how the change occurred during the Reagan administration. Initially, Mr. Reagan referred to the Russians as "the evil empire" and "the enemy." A few years later, news photos showed Reagan with his arm around Gorbachev proclaiming them great friends.

Gorbachev related the initial negotiations between him and Reagan were based on the United States telling Gorbachev how his country should be run. Gorbachev was a great negotiator as well as a great thinker. Over the course of these talks, he began shaping a new view of this relationship. He told Reagan he wanted to move toward a point where the United States needed Russia. He said it was important the United States and its economy become dependent on Russia. He further related he wished Russia to become dependent both economically and philosophically on the United States. It was his feeling if both countries depended on each other, neither would ever push the button and begin a nuclear war. Each would also have a greater need to continue and nurture the relationship. This was obviously a successful plan. We have seen the demise of Communism in Russia and truly the beginning of the relationship he described. This paradigm shift changed not only our countries' relationships but much of the nature of the European community.

As stated in a previous chapter, the unfortunate inaccurate accepted paradigm today is most people with nerve problems have carpal tunnel. This leads to narrow thinking and does not allow treatment and cures for patients who fall outside the generally accepted norms. It also belittles many of the often helpful alternative treatments and methods of healing. The onus of responsibility is the patient's; to either respond to standard accepted cures or accept the responsibility for failure as their own. The basis of the paradigm is patients who have nerve problems have carpal tunnel and if they do not improve with simple surgery, there is a problem with the patient. It's obvious this is a self-fulfilling defeatist prophecy.

Robbins goes on to say people who are successful in this world are able to see beyond the standard accepted views of problems. They have an ability to change their paradigm or orientation as to the way they think about life or disease. Eventually these people change the paradigms of others, and this is when they become successful. They are able to view their problems from more than one aspect by stepping outside the accepted vantage point. With this understanding of nerve disease, alternative treatments and philosophies become not only acceptable but vital in the healing process.

Here's a true story of something that happened to my dad years ago. One morning he awakened with a severely swollen painful right wrist. His immediate visit to the family practitioner resulted in an X-ray taken with an antiquated yet functional piece of equipment. The conclusion was "a build-up of calcium deposit touching a nerve" (actually, it was a ganglion cyst, a fluid-filled sac coming from the wrist joint). He was sent to a radiologist who took further films and declared the diagnosis "correct." The radiologist told my father to come back the next day and it would be dissolved with X-rays.

My dad phoned his family doctor again and was advised to see a local surgeon before going back to the X-ray suite. The surgeon also confirmed the diagnosis as "correct." He concluded by stating, "See you tomorrow and we will remove this surgically before it gets worse."

My dad wisely went back to his family practitioner. As they talked, his doctor held a large medical text and read to him. His doctor went to reach for his hand and my dad involuntarily withdrew his arm in pain. He gently placed my dad's hand back on the desk and suddenly without warning slammed the text down on top of his hand impacting directly at the most tender point. My dad's anguished hollering of "What the heck are you doing?" was met by a sly smile from his doctor. He said he was simply "breaking up the calcium deposit." Two days later, the swelling resolved and the cyst was gone.

Each of these physicians was absolutely correct in his diagnosis and each treatment regimen recommended was appropriate. Each of them was taught by specialist trainers to deal with the problem in his own way. The family practitioner drew upon his years of experience and recognized a more simplistic approach to the problem. This was the perfect example of versatility, open-mindedness, and a broad knowledge base.

There is a caveat to the above story. In the classic description of this incident, the physician used a Bible, not a text. One of my patients had heard a similar story about breaking up a ganglion cyst using a Bible. He felt if the Bible was good, the unabridged dictionary would be better. He tried this on his wife. Unfortunately, the cyst did not rupture but he was successful in breaking her wrist. Perhaps our medical training only teaches us better aim!

In patients with complex nerve problems and pain, there is a very strong emotional and stress-related aspect to physical pain. If a patient can control or at least decrease stress, he or she can often obtain good relief from symptomatology.

There are two factors about nerves that make this scenario predictable. The first is nerves run through muscular beds, which means nerves run between layers of muscle. Muscles work by either contracting or relaxing. When we are stressed, muscles become tighter and more tense. What happens when these muscles contract is they essentially press or squeeze the nerves running between them. When there is compression of these nerves, this causes symptoms in the way of pain, discomfort, and numbness.

The second issue concerning nerves is they all have their own intrinsic blood supply. This means aside from the blood vessels that run throughout our body, nerves have their own separate circulation, which is actually inside the structure of the nerve. Further, all arteries have muscle tissue in their walls and the ability to constrict or expand, thus decreasing or increasing blood flow. When nerves and their accompanying blood vessels become scarred or abnormally stressed, the spasm causes constriction and reduction of this blood flow; the result is less nutrition and oxygen flows to the nerves. In the short term, this may result in minor discomfort. When this happens over a long period of time, the result is chronic disability manifesting as pain, numbness, spasticity, increased sensitivity, cold intolerance, and so forth.

It should now be clear the previous scenario can lead to both short- and long-term problems. Negative emotions such as anxiety, depression, anger, and stress can have significant and deleterious effects on the nervous system. It is essential the physician consider the degree of anxiety, depression, stress, and other related issues that go along with nerve problems. It is here the open-mindedness of the physician as well as the patient constitute the essential ingredients for these alternative treatments work.

"Tim" was a patient who had significant carpal tunnel involvement and substantial tendinitis with pain in his arms. He had not been successful in relieving his symptoms with standard treatment in the way of therapy and medications. His tendinitis and inflammatory disease exacerbated his nerve pain and his fingers actually locked down and he was unable to open his hand on many days.

Tim was told there was absolutely nothing that could be done for him; he had a pain syndrome and surgery would make him worse rather than better. Consequently, he was not allowed to have surgery, but he could not get better by standard nonsurgical methods. We had no choice but to find alternative treatments for him. Even if I did recommend surgery, we would not be able to obtain approval.

It has been many years now and although he has never cured his problem, he has modified his life substantially. As a machinist and inventor, he built himself an entire home therapy unit, including a heated whirlpool. Through his own home remedies and good sense, he has been able to live with significant disease. Perhaps he has actually done better through his modifications than he would have if he had gone ahead with standard protocols and surgery.

For thousands of years, Far Eastern cultures, medicine, and philosophy have taught peace, serenity, relaxation, and oneness with the environment are essential in the healing process. Unfortunately, the philosophy of the Western world is stress, lack of free time, and constant striving are admirable qualities. Meditation, gentleness, and relaxation are equated with laziness and weakness.

I believe the term "work ethic" has been mislabeled. Perhaps it should be more appropriately called "work effect." We are taught from the time we are very young we must achieve, produce, and continue to work. In the United States, the more work we do, the harder we work, and the sicker we become both emotionally and physically, the better person we are labeled. We are taught to make as much money as we can, then spend it to the point where we don't have enough to maintain our lifestyle. We then work even harder. This is an interesting phenomenon and unfortunately quite pathologic. We become caught in a cycle of continuing work and harming ourselves, a sort of psychological cumulative trauma disorder. The only real way out is to become so sick we must stop. Proper balance between work, play, pleasure, and pain must be achieved. Although this balance does not come easily, once we achieve it, our lives become happier and healthier.

"Victor" has achieved such balance. Injured in a serious car accident, Victor broke his wrist badly and sustained significant injury to his shoulders. He has underlying nerve problems with numbness, but his main issue has been pain and disability. By profession, Victor is a bridge painter and also a slight-of-hand artist. I have seen Victor's magic and I know his medical problems. He continues to amaze me at his wonderful agility with respect to his hands and arms in spite of his injuries.

What balances Victor is that his magic and sleight of hand are the best therapy he could have. This has helped him with mobility and balances his pain with pleasure. This is a man who loves what he does. Through his own personal magic, he has made a potentially untenable and unlivable situation more than tolerable. He has gone back to his regular job as a bridge painter and has maintained homeostasis in severely problematic arms by the use of his own healing powers. He has combined work, play, and pleasure into a true healing process.

We are rarely taught to relax, but undoubtedly, each and every one of us knows how to become stressed at the drop of a hat. Stress is the norm—accepted and recognized as part of our daily living routine. Only recently has medicine re-evolved to the point where we are recognizing that the use of relaxation techniques in the way of biofeedback, hypnosis, meditation, yoga, and *tai chi* are not only useful but possibly essential in healing. Experience has shown us many patients use these adjunctive techniques and get relief from these "supplementary modalities." In fact, many are able to overcome their problems and actually reverse their physiologic changes and nerve conduction studies by incorporating these techniques into their daily lives and activities.

There are those who doubt the benefits of hypnosis and biofeedback and call them hocus-pocus or "magical wishful thinking." It is, however, well documented that physiologic changes do occur with the use of biofeedback and relaxation techniques. Biofeedback itself has been used for many years to help patients with a wide variety of medical disorders including Raynaud's syndrome. This is a problem caused by spasm or constriction of the blood vessels; when exposed to cold, the fingers can actually turn blue or white. It is often a very painful condition and some patients have even lost fingers and toes because of this disease. Using biofeedback, patients are actually able to increase blood flow to their digits and decrease their reactivity to cold exposures. This generally results in decreased pain and symptoms.

"George" came to me after he sustained a severe injury to his left hand. He was a farmer and had a crush injury to his hand by a plow shear. He already had an amputation of one finger, and there were significant problems with lack of ability to move his hand and his other digits. He also had substantial pain and problems with cold intolerance as well as severe nerve involvement. Because of the crush as well as a traction (yanking) injury to the extremity, he had significant involvement with the nerves at multiple levels in his hand and arm including his median nerve at the wrist and brachial plexus. His problems included severe cold intolerance (pain with exposure to cold environments), and the temperature in his hand was well below normal limits for circulation and temperature curves.

Because of his severe pain, we decided to give George a trial of biofeedback and relaxation techniques. With these procedures, not only was George able to raise the temperature of his hand close to 18 degrees at will, but he was actually able to eliminate his pain and symptoms. We were able to avoid surgical procedures for nerve decompression at all levels. Today this strong-willed man is able to continue work and has had remarkable ability to utilize his biofeedback and relaxation techniques for pain management. He has decreased his symptoms to the point where he is able to live productively with this severely disabled extremity.

Now that we've established these adjunctive therapies as desirable and at times essential in the healing process, there are other factors that need to be discussed. The first is the problem of time and rapport. None of these techniques can be learned without the physician and patient taking the time to understand the principles behind them. It is further necessary to establish an ability to use the technique. Trust as well as an adequate rapport between patient and physician is essential for this to occur.

In today's world of managed care, the emphasis is not on quality of care but rather quantity. There is tremendous pressure on health practitioners today to see as many patients as possible and do this "efficiently." This does not allow doctors time to get to know their patients and determine which would be able to utilize these techniques or be willing. After making the decision that these techniques would be helpful, there comes the further need for approval from health care organizations, many of which feel that techniques with a 70 percent success rate are not "financially wise." Once we've gotten past these hurdles, there comes the necessity for the healer as well as the patient to take the time out of their schedules to actually teach and learn these techniques. It must be emphasized appropriate selection of the patient is imperative to match the technique to the patient. For example, a person who cannot sit still would not be a good candidate for meditation or relaxation techniques but might indeed benefit from an exercise program or *tai chi*–type protocol with the goal of relaxation through motion. Only a trained professional and someone very familiar with these adjunctive modalities can help determine exactly which would be right for a particular patient and allow appropriate utilization.

"Jerry" was involved in severe motor vehicle accident. He sustained injury to the nerves of his brachial plexus and a left wrist injury with nerve as well as ligament involvement. Jerry is a highly successful insurance executive whose job consisted of a substantial amount of driving. He had ample stress in his life and after this devastating injury, he was forced to put many things on hold.

Jerry undertook our treatment program with a vengeance. His day began at 5:00 A.M. and incorporated morning prayer with his biofeedback pain management techniques. He undertook a walking program as well as exercising five days a week, including stair climber, treadmill, and low-level weights. He changed the way he worked by becoming a managing supervisor. He stopped driving, letting the people he was working with and training drive him around instead.

Today Jerry's arm is not normal, but he has taken an understanding of his disease and approached curing himself with as much time, energy, and effort as possible. This has paid off handsomely. He is greatly improved and functioning close to his previous capacities.

This is not to say his disease is gone. Jerry still has significant underlying disease but he knows how to control it. When he goes outside of his limitations, he notes exacerbations and increased symptoms. On the other hand, when he stays within his limits, he has made himself pain free. This is not a person I have cured. He is someone who, through understanding how to manage his pain and nerve injuries, has made his life close to normal once again. He notes other benefits to himself and his life from these changes spiritually.

With respect to alternative treatments, many people who are not truly qualified call themselves healers and experts. These range from "quacks" to well-meaning laypeople who are utilizing techniques improperly. People who teach biofeedback techniques and yoga or use hypnosis and other ancillary treatments need to be well qualified and licensed in these areas. If this is not the case, these techniques may not work and may even be harmful. Let your treating physician and/or family doctor help you locate people who are qualified.

The goal of biofeedback and relaxation techniques is to decrease our sympathetically mediated response to daily stresses and stimuli. (Dr. Herbert Benson in his book *Beyond the Relaxation Response* termed this the "relaxation response" and describes many of the physiologic issues involved.) This training is not greatly different from that used to teach secret service agents or undercover people to react immediately to stimuli and dangers. Their responses are quick and predictable. This is no different than the boxer or martial artist, with skills honed to the point where reflexes take over before fear and immobilization can inhibit a response.

With time and practice, these techniques become a part of our psyche. When stress causes increased spasm and decreased blood flow, our new reaction becomes one of releasing that stress and inducing a relaxation or healing response. Once these techniques are learned in the presence of the healer, many of them can and should be practiced and thus intensified. They can be of tremendous value when learned and applied appropriately. In our experience, relaxation techniques and behavior modification are often enough to keep patients out of the operating room and free of pain.

Alternatives
and the Future

CHAPTER 13

*"You gain strength, courage and
confidence by every experience in which
you really stop to look fear in the face.
You are able to say to yourself,
'I lived through this horror. I can take
the next thing that comes along....'
You must do the thing
you think you cannot do."*

—Anna Eleanor Roosevelt

It is my hope you now realize nerve problems are complex yet simple. Treating a nerve problem is no different than finding the right mate, career, or exercise regimen. Incorporated in this process is a good deal of planning, soul searching, and obtaining the best possible education you can to allow yourself to make appropriate decisions. What becomes obvious is what the process really requires is a desire to heal and get better and a commitment to proceed on these lines. That commitment must come out of a well-formed relationship between patient and healer.

There is no doubt there are people who, no matter how aggressively conservative treatment is undertaken, will require surgery. Indeed many have surgery and do well. There are others who have surgery and do not do so well. The majority of patients, however, do only as well as their understanding of their disease allows. Although most people improve with conservative or surgical treatment, people with nerve problems rarely become "normal" again. What is necessary is a realistic understanding of the expectations from any treatment. Once each of us understands exactly what we are trying to achieve with a treatment program or protocol, the results are no doubt better from both a mental and a physiologic point of view.

Sometimes understanding the relationship is essential when people don't get better. "Sarah" was stable and doing fairly well at calming her severe pain syndrome and multiple-level nerve problem. Although surgery had given her some relief, it was incomplete. We were looking at the possibility of a second and third surgery at her elbow and brachial plexus level because she told me she was having a significant exacerbation of her symptoms.

I was lucky enough to have a trusting relationship with Sarah and I was able to gain a little better understanding of her home life. It seems Sarah had exacerbated her symptoms because she had been sleeping on the floor. When I questioned why, she related she had not been able to sleep in her house for some time and had been sleeping at a relative's. She explained someone had missed a turn and driven a car right into her dining room, literally. The car remained in her dining room, displacing her table. The entire front of her apartment was exposed to the cold. Luckily no one was injured directly, but Sarah's stress level as well as home life had been disrupted. There were some insurance entanglements and no one was removing the car. This series of events significantly exacerbated her upper extremity problems and her pain symptoms.

I am happy to report the car is out of Sarah's dining room. We were able to move forward with her second surgery from which she got excellent relief at her elbow level and her thoracic outlet. We've found it is often imperative to stabilize a person's home situation before we can hope to get relief. This applies to conservative as well as operative and perioperative (the time before and after a surgery) care. A relaxed and happy mind helps a body heal.

I would like to mention a word or two about vitamins and nutrition therapy. There has been a good deal of research concerning the healing of nerves and the use of the B-complex vitamins in nerve healing. There is some compelling evidence to indicate nerve regeneration and self-repair is helped by B-complex vitamins. Appropriate doses are not an unreasonable avenue to try. I have not personally seen anyone cured by taking B-complex vitamins alone but I have rarely seen anyone harmed either. They are utilized by nerves in the regeneration process and adequate supplies are needed. As part of an overall well-developed regimen with exercise, modification of lifestyle, and conservative as well as possible surgical treatment, this is a good adjunct and is certainly worth trying.

Antioxidants such as vitamins C and E are getting a lot of press today as well. It is apparent they are helpful in the treatment of medical problems in general and the process of healing. These are believed to work by binding up "free radicals," which are tiny little scavengers in our bodies presumed to do damage to tissues. On the basis of forming healthier scar tissue and allowing better regeneration with less problems, these seem a reasonable addition to any healing program. I recommend any patient wishing to begin vitamin or modified nutrition therapy should consult his or her family practitioner prior to undertaking this to be sure of the appropriate doses.

"Jenna" worked as a psychiatric hospital security aide and sustained a substantial injury when she was attacked by a patient. She sustained severe injury to her left thumb and arm. She ultimately required surgery for median nerve decompression and was diagnosed as having a substantial brachial plexus problem on the left.

It became apparent early in Jenna's treatment she would not be able to return to her previous job as a psych security aide. She managed to control her pain through her biofeedback techniques and heal with the use of vitamins. Jenna decided to go back to school. She is soon to complete her degree as a dietician. Although her arm is not normal, she obtained good enough relief to keep her from requiring high risk operative intervention. Jenna is a wonderful example of someone who has taken a negative situation and turned apparent bad luck into opportunity.

I'm a strong personal believer in exercise on a regular basis. There is no doubt the increase in circulation and blood flow to nerves as well as muscles, joints, and ligaments maintains their elasticity and ability to function. Many patients who have pain for a period of time or undergo multiple surgeries and treatments become deconditioned. They are forced into basically sedentary lifestyles and are not able to perform the daily and regular activities they did previously. Many patients go from very active to completely sedentary lifestyles under our direction. We have become much more aware today of the need to keep patients moving. Indeed women used to be kept in the hospital for a week or longer after delivering babies and asked to stay at bed rest. Many medical problems ensued secondary to this. In orthopedics, we have found the earlier we begin motion post-operatively, the better the result and the less problems we have with stiffness, joint restriction, and even loss of bone density. This applies to many surgeries from joint replacements to nerve repair.

As Gandhi said, "A person cannot do right in one department of life whilst attempting to do wrong in another department. Life is one indivisible whole." This applies to our mind-body relationship. An entire program of "right" things from physical to metaphysical must be tailored to each person. As long as these are well founded physiologically and emotionally—you will heal.

The type of exercise performed does not really seem to matter as long as there is a regular routine enjoyable to you as an individual. Exercise does not necessarily need to be aggressive but it must be aerobic to some extent. Let's differentiate aerobic exercises from bulking or weight lifting. There are people who enjoy weight lifting and believe toning their muscles and gaining bulk is helpful. Excessive bulking and strengthening are only helpful to people who are exposed to environments with stresses above and beyond those expected from daily living. If, for example, you lift 200-pound boxes regularly for a living or wrestle with linebackers, then developing your upper body musculature is reasonable. On the other hand, if you push a pen all day long and the heaviest thing you lift is your baby, then bulking and conditioning to lift 200 pounds at a time is not only unnecessary but often counter-productive. The increased bulk and stress on muscles can sometimes be as detrimental as helpful.

There are some therapy programs based on aggressive conditioning and strengthening with aggressive upper body exercise. Many promote the "no pain, no gain" theory. I warn my patients against these type programs. If weights are to be incorporated, they should be light weights and only at regular limited intervals, building slowly. The use of free weight puts significant stress on joint, muscle, ligament, and nerve tissues. Essentially they are at the end of a long lever, and

175

these weights put significant traction on the proximal extremity where the nerves originate.

Recommended exercises include anything from mild aerobic activities such as tennis, basketball, aerobics, or karate, to dance and *tai chi,* which is described as "meditation in motion." Even patients with severe limitations and disabilities are candidates for some type of program; walking is an excellent exercise. I particularly like swimming and if not formal swimming, at least getting in the water and moving around. This eliminates gravity as a stress issue and allows a stress-free environment. One caution about walking and swimming is the upper arm swing may be stressful, especially with problems such as thoracic outlet syndrome. I recommend walking with your hands in your pockets with a light windbreaker or swimming where overhead crawl strokes are avoided. Each person obviously is individual and needs to find the activities that do not bother him or her. The basic rule of thumb is if it feels good, go ahead and do it. If you are actually feeling better after doing these exercises, then they are right for you.

I think we've made it quite clear appropriate meditation and relaxation techniques should be incorporated in everyone's regimen. There is no doubt reduction of overall stress in our lives makes people feel better. We all feel better when we are happy and worse when we are sad. We are better when loving than when being angry. This is more than just a feeling but rather based on the physiologic release of endorphins and enkephalins as well as increasing or decreasing muscle spasm. There are many good techniques for relaxing and we've mentioned only a few in this book. Suffice it to say, find the one which is right for you.

Stephen Covey relates a wonderful story in the beginning of his book, *The Seven Habits of Highly Successful People.* He talks about the process of co-dependency and the nature of interpersonal relationships. He described one of his sons who was, by his estimation, not very good at anything. He had problems with playing ball, school, relationships, and basically anything he attempted to master. An extreme co-dependent relationship developed between child and parents. Dr. Covey found he was constantly protecting this child, making excuses for him, and supporting him with respect to his relationships with the other children and also in all avenues of his life.

What he eventually discovered was the problem was not with his son but with his own attitude toward his son, which was based on the "assumption" anything his son tried he would fail. This became, in a bizarre sense, his son's only way of obtaining approval, love, and cooperation from his parents. Dr. Covey was wise enough to recognize this. He changed his own paradigm or way of looking at his son; he allowed him to succeed or fail on his own. In response, his son became highly successful and subsequently changed his behavior. He sought not failure for approval but sought success instead.

We find this type of relationship with many patients today. The system rewards people both financially and at times with sympathy and recognition for having disease and pain. There are even a few who focus their whole lives around nurturing, fostering, and living through their disabilities. Their disability becomes their identity. Others are caught in a system that punishes them for attempting to return to even modified work activities. The system often attempts to force people back into the environments and situations that injured them in the first place. This sets up a dangerous scenario and vicious cycle.

One man I recall worked in a paper mill. His hand and arm were sucked into a milling machine. He was pinned in the machine for almost an hour. He underwent a significant

177

amount of therapy to stabilize him physically and psychologically. He was understandably hesitant to go back to the same job. Instead of finding him alternative employment, his employer insisted he return to this mill and this machine. Needless to say he refused, wisely, and found employment elsewhere. Others are not so lucky.

We must remember pain is a positive. Pain tells us there is something wrong. It is a warning sign from our body something needs to change. As long as both the healer and patient recognize pain is a good thing, it can become part of the healing process. Positive results will no doubt follow.

So where do you go from here? This book is perhaps a starting point for you on your road to recovery. The thoughts, ideas, and concepts in this book are truly only one man's opinion. Yes, they are based on years of training and the teachings of many others I've incorporated into my own personal healing and treatment style. The information is based on my experience with thousands of patients who have followed these scriptions and healed. Much of what I am relating here has been taught to me by my patients and I thank them all for this.

You have basically been armed with a plan and an understanding of where that plan comes from. It is now up to you to take this information and apply it to yourself and assemble an appropriate team to help you heal. Remember, no one knows you, your body, or your disease better than you. It is simply formulating your own understanding of the disease that is necessary and then applying the appropriate treatments from people you can communicate with, who understand you, and most importantly, in whom you trust.

Do not allow your body or sensibility to be violated by the constraints of the new medicine and the economics of managed care. Once you understand what you need, you will be able to seek it out. Remember, it is your job to tell your doctor where you need to go and what type of treatment you need. As long as he or she understands your explanation, they should be able to direct you appropriately. If they can't, you need a new doctor and a new plan.

GLOSSARY

Adson's Test

This test is performed by having the patient turn his or her head to the right or left while holding the arms either up and away from the body or down and away from center line while the examiner checks the pulse. This test is done to evaluate the vascular status of a brachial plexus problem. It is meant only to evaluate for circulatory problems which will be helpful in diagnosing vascular thoracic outlet problems. It's important to note that only approximately three to five percent of patients with thoracic outlet problems have "vascular involvement".

Alternative Medicine

A general term describing multiple techniques such as acupuncture, massage therapy, hypno-therapy, biofeedback, manipulative therapy, and the like. It is used to indicate treatments not generally accepted as part of "standard medical practice." It has gained great respect in recent years due to validation of its successes and more public awareness that many standard medical treatments are not as successful as previously thought.

Anterior Scalene Muscle

This is the front of a group of three muscles in the neck through which the nerves of the brachial plexus travel. During thoracic outlet surgery, the anterior scalene muscle may be cut or removed to help treat the pathology.

Artery

Tubes of many sizes lined by muscle which travel through the body bringing blood away from the heart. Arteries have the ability to constrict (close down), thereby decreasing the amount of blood flow, or dilate (open wider), increasing the blood flow to an area, in either normal or pathologic states.

Arthroscopic Surgery

See Endoscopic Surgery.

Axon

The cell body or primary control center of a nerve.

Behavior Modification

Change in the patterns of a patient's daily living. This may include utilization of relaxation techniques as well as a regular exercise program. It often includes modification in the way patients perform activities, changes in posture, use of body mechanics, and altering the way the patient utilizes their body. A technique in which the physician, therapist, and patient identify activities which are harmful to that patient and then change the way these activities are performed or eliminate them from a patient's lifestyle.

Biofeedback

A technique utilized in the management of pain and many vascular and nerve diseases. A relaxation technique where patients are taught deep breathing exercises and learn to relax muscles and increase blood flow. The patient is essentially given "feedback", either visually on a monitor or by auditory input. This is a painless therapy modality which requires active participation of the patient but can be utilized while outside the therapy unit.

Brachial Plexus

The anatomic term describing all of the nerves that travel between the neck and shoulder which become the major nerves in the arm. They travel through a tunnel or channel called the thoracic outlet.

Carpal bones

Eight bones of the wrist which move and rotate around each other to allow rotatory motion of the wrist. They form the floor of the carpal canal at the carpal tunnel level.

Carpal Tunnel Syndrome

A generalized term used to describe symptoms in the upper extremities. Originally it described a very limited set of symptoms which indicated median nerve involvement only at the wrist level. It is hallmarked by numbness and tingling in the thumb, index, long, and radial half of the ring finger. Patients often have pain and discomfort which classically awakens them at night.

Conservative Care

Refers to treatment in a nonoperative and non-invasive realm. This includes therapy, lifestyle modification, biofeedback relaxation techniques, manipulation, and alternative medicine treatments.

Cubital Tunnel

The groove on the inside of the elbow through which the ulnar nerve (the funny bone nerve) travels. Problems here may cause numbness and tingling in the small and ring finger and weakness in the hand.

Cumulative Trauma Disorder

Also known as repetitive stress syndrome, overuse syndrome, or repetitive trauma. This pathologic entity is marked by multiple and repeated minor insults to an extremity which result in inflammation and, subsequently, scarring about the nerve, tendon, and muscle structures. Over a prolonged period of time, repeated minor insults—such as keying, hammering, repetitive reaching, and the like—result in pathology which becomes fixed and produces long-term disabling symptomatology.

Decompression

Freeing a nerve from pressure. For example, releasing a ligament at the carpal tunnel or a band of muscle at the level of the thoracic outlet. At times, more than simply a decompression may be necessary to give relief from nerve problems especially if there is severe scarring about the nerve.

Dendrite

The long tentacle-like structure of a nerve which carries impulses from the axon or main body to another nerve or its end point.

Depression

A state which ensues for various reasons where patients are less reactive and inter-active with the world. Depression may be a chemically-mediated problem which occurs for no reason, or may be a reactive issue which occurs in response to a specific situation. The latter usually resolves once the stress or pressure is removed from the individual.

Diagnosis

A basic working premise a physician uses when formulating an overall treatment plan for disease. The diagnosis is based on history as well as examination and diagnostic tests. Initial diagnoses can be changed if the facts and test results warrant.

Dislocation

A process which occurs where the bones of a joint are traumatized and displaced from their normal anatomic position. This may occur at the level of the carpal tunnel where most commonly the lunate (one of the carpal bones) may dislocate and be pushed into the carpal tunnel. This may result in symptoms of numbness, tingling, and pain.

Double Crush

Can describe more than one level of nerve involvement in an extremity. A classic example is a patient with a herniated disc at the neck as well as carpal tunnel involvement. These patients have more than one area of pressure on a specific nerve and will often get incomplete or no relief when they have surgery or conservative treatment at one level only.

Dupuytren's

An abnormal thickening of the tissues of the lining of the palm. This is hallmarked by a progressive, very often slow contracting of these tissues, which may pull the fingers down into the palm in a fixed position. It is generally treated with surgical intervention. Patients with Dupuytren's have a higher risk of developing reflex sympathetic dystrophy with surgery than the general population. Its cause is essentially unknown.

Dysesthesias

A medical term used to describe altered sensations. These may be in the form of numbness, tingling, coldness, burning, throbbing, stabbing, or pain. Refers to the grouping indicating altered sensibility.

Edema

Swelling in an area.

Electromyelography/Nerve Conduction Velocity Testing

Testing performed by either inserting a needle or placing an electrode on an extremity. A recording sensor is then placed at another portion of the extremity. The nerve is then pulsed with an electrical impulse and a determination as to that nerve's capability to conduct electricity is made. This testing is done to isolate nerve pathology. This is a very examiner-dependent test and a negative study does not always indicate that pathology is not present.

Endoscopic Surgery

Surgery done with the use of a endoscope or arthroscope. These instruments are essentially very small telescopes attached to cameras. They have a light source and are often confused with "laser" instruments. Essentially the light is only for viewing. Through arthroscopic surgery, techniques can be performed with more limited incisions. Many times endoscopic or arthroscopic surgery can be performed allowing the same type operation or a more limited operation to be done with smaller incisions and less trauma. There is a high learning curve for surgeons to perfect these techniques.

Epineurium

The outer layer or lining of a nerve proper. The sheath in which the nerve fibers or fascicles travel.

Exercise

Any regularly performed activity which allows us to increase our heart rate and help tone our muscles. Ideally, this should incorporate aerobic as well as toning and stretching routines to allow not only maintenance of muscular function but also the heart and vascular system.

Fracture

A broken bone.

Hand Surgeon

A surgeon specifically trained in diagnosis and conservative as well as operative treatment of upper extremity problems. This physician has training above and beyond the general expertise expected of an orthopaedic or plastic surgeon; generally in the way of a fellowship which is extended training after residency has been completed.

Healing

The process by which an organism recovers from an injury. This may be on the basis of decrease in inflammation or mend-

186

ing of torn or stretched structures. When structures are damaged, most heal by the formation of scar tissue except bones which heal by the formation of new bone.

Herniated Disc

This is a misunderstood term. Discs are essentially spacers or cushions present between the bones of the spine or the vertebrae. Discs may be injured when their thickened outer liner (the annulus fibrosis) is torn or injured. The inner softer substance (nucleus pulposus) pushes out of its normal contained environment. In a true herniated disc, the nucleus pulposus extrudes or comes out of its sac and may press on a nerve root or the spinal cord itself causing nerve symptoms. Very often patients will have a bulge in a disc where there is simply some weakening of the thick annulus fibrosis. The bulge does not generally cause symptoms. Unfortunately, many people interchangeably use the terms disc bulge and disc herniation. They are very different with respect to treatment and diagnostic ramifications.

History

A discussion which takes place between physician and patient. This includes the details of the patient's problem and also the mechanism by which it occurred.

Hunter Test

A test performed by having a patient bring his or her arms up and away from the body (the "stick 'em up" position) or down and behind the body with various wrist postures. If a reproduction of nerve symptoms occur, this indicates pathology at the level of the thoracic outlet.

Inflammation

Swelling of soft tissues in the body. Most often associated with the lining structures of joints such as the synovium or the surrounding lining of nerves or tendons as in the epineurium or tenosynovium. When present, this is usually accompanied by fullness or swelling and often results in pain.

Injections

Using a needle to administer substances to either decrease pain or inflammation. When used appropriately, these may be helpful in calming down inflammatory processes.

Keloid

A very thick and unsightly scar which forms at times in certain patients. Keloid scars are indicative of aggressive scar formation in individuals and may indicate that these patients have a tendency toward aggressive or thicker scar formation which may result in less than ideal results with surgery.

Leeches

Small animals which are parasitic in nature and survive by attaching to a host who they draw blood from. They have been used medically for many years in various ways. They are currently utilized to help replanted digits survive when they become congested or filled with blood due to inadequate return circulation.

Lifestyle Modification

Similar to behavior modification. A change in the way people go about their daily activities. This may incorporate meditation techniques to decrease stress, increase in exercise, or change in diet. Hopefully it is a positive change made to live within the limitations of one's disease.

Managed Care

A type of insurance whereby gatekeepers control the flow and delivery of medical care. Patients need to go through specific channels and proper levels of authority to obtain more intensive medical care and treatment.

Manipulation

This may be in the form of osteopathic manipulation or chiropractic manipulation or adjustments. There are many techniques utilized today to re-align or re-adjust the tissues of the spine and/or at times the extremities. This is often helpful in decreasing muscle spasm and relieving the pain and discomfort of nerve problems.

Massage Therapy

Therapy performed by rubbing or kneading the tissues in various manners. Trained massage therapists are often able to decrease muscle spasm and thereby decrease nerve pain.

Median Nerve

The nerve which begins at the fifth and sixth nerve roots at the neck and travels down through the arm into the carpal tunnel. This supplies feeling to the thumb, index, long fingers, and thumb side of the ring finger. It also supplies the thenar muscles to the thumb.

Mesoepineurium

The fine cobweb-like normal scar tissue which surrounds nerves and holds them in place. When traumatized, this very fine lining may become inflamed and thickened resulting in some types of nerve pathology.

Mobilization

A term used in surgery to indicate freeing of a nerve or structure from surrounding scar tissue or compression. It indicates the nerve has been freed so it is allowed to move or glide freely through its surrounding tissue beds.

Motor Nerve

A nerve which conducts impulses from the brain and spinal cord to the extremities. This impulse tells a muscle to contract, resulting in motion and/or motor function.

MRI (Magnetic Resonance Imaging)

MRI scanners utilize a magnetic field and computer to reproduce images of soft tissue structures within the body. They allow discs as well as nerve and spinal cord structures to be seen. They do not, though, tell us how these structures are functioning. They simply give an image of these structures and allow us to rule in or out various types of pathology with respect to the structural integrity or abnormality of these tissues.

Multi-Level Neuropathy

A term used to indicate more than one level or area in an extremity being involved with pathology and/or scar tissue resulting in nerve problems. When patients have multi-level nerve disease, they often get incomplete relief from treatment and/or surgery aimed at only one level of the nerve disease. (see Double Crush)

Nerve Block

Injections performed usually at the level of the neck or thoracic outlet. These are, at times, helpful in decreasing pain and sympathetic reactivity in patients who have failed to respond to conservative care. They are not without risk and carry the possibility of damage to nerve structures as well as the structures of the thorax.

Nerves

Structures which are anatomically threaded throughout the body varying in diameter from a large pen to less than a millimeter. These structures carry electrical impulses and are responsible for allowing sensation as well as controlling muscles.

Nonsteroidal Anti-Inflammatory Medication (NSAIDs)

Medications taken to decrease inflammation in the body. Common brands are Motrin, Naprosyn, Feldene, Clinoril, and Indocin to name a few. They help in controlling pain as well as decreasing inflammation. They do have a number of side effects including stomach upset and the possibility of bleeding problems. They should be used with care but are quite effective in many problems where inflammation is the major issue.

Numbness

A term which in its absolute sense means no feeling. This term is often misused by patients and physicians to indicate altered sensation or a "not normal feeling."

Nutrition

The study of mineral & vitamin intake and dietary needs of the body. It is acknowledged today that nutrition plays a vital role in the body's ability to heal and maintain itself properly.

Pain

The body's natural way of telling us that something is wrong. An indication of pathology in an area and to stop doing whatever is causing the discomfort. If pain is unrelenting, it may require treatment.

Pain Syndrome

Describes patients who have pain where there is not a specific cause or etiology for the same. Pain syndromes are hallmarked by severe pain, discomfort, and disability without a treatable cause.

Paradigm

An accepted belief system or way of thinking. Paradigms are based on standard accepted ideas, concepts, and personal experiences. They are changeable.

Pathology

Disease. Abnormalities in the body which are found and are consistent with a disease process.

Perception

An accepted viewpoint based on a person's understanding of a problem or issue. This may be correct or incorrect and valid or not valid, depending on what information is available and how we are able to incorporate it.

Phalen's Test

A test performed by asking the patient to bend the wrists in the reverse of the prayer position and hold this posture for sixty seconds. If a reproduction of nerve symptoms in either the median or ulnar nerve distribution is present, this may indicate pathology of the median or ulnar nerve at the wrist or hand level.

Physical Examination

That portion of an evaluation by a physician which incorporates the laying on of hands performing various tests to determine the nature of the pathology and to help delineate the exact level of disease. This should be performed on an entire extremity and not just at the area of the obvious pathology. (i.e. from neck to fingertips)

Physical or Occupational Therapy

Incorporates the application of various modalities in the way of heat, ice, or modalities such as ultrasound, iontophoresis, hot packs, and TENS units. This also incorporates various exercises and hands-on manipulations or massage techniques to give patients relief from their pain and symptomatology. Therapy is done in many ways and a basic rule of thumb is that it should help to improve symptoms and should not be painful.

Physician

By definition, a healer. A person trained in either osteopathic, allopathic, or homeopathic methods to name a few. They have the ability to utilize conservative care as well as medications and surgery when necessary to treat and hopefully heal disease.

Radial Nerve

This nerve begins at the C-7 nerve root in the neck and travels down through the arm on the outside of the elbow and continues to supply sensation to the back side of the hand.

This nerve allows wrist extension and straightening of the fingers.

Radiograph (X-ray)

A study done to evaluate the integrity and structure of the bone(s). We may see, at times, foreign bodies or inflammation in the soft tissues. It will not show anything about the structure, integrity or function of the nerves or muscles.

Recurrence

Disease which comes back after it is resolved or improved with treatment. With respect to nerve problems, this is generally caused by renewed inflammation or progressive formation of the scar tissue about nerve structures.

Reflex Sympathetic Dystrophy

A phenomenon which occurs when the sympathetic nerves, which travel from the neck through the brachial plexus into the arm, become over-activated. It is hallmarked by severe pain, often with color changes in the extremity and severe disability. It is often described as pain out of proportion to the nature of the injury.

Repetitive

Something that is done on a repeated basis.

Risk

A term which indicates the possibility of problems after undertaking an intervention. There are risks to most treatments and the more aggressive the treatment, the more substantial the possible risks. These should be understood by anyone before undertaking a treatment.

Roos test

This test is performed by having the patient bring his or her arms up above the head and slightly away from center line. If holding this position for sixty seconds or longer reproduces nerve symptoms, this may indicate pathology at the level of brachial plexus.

Scar

The tissue our body forms to replace torn or damaged structures. It is the body's normal repair material.

Sensory Nerve

A nerve which conducts electrical impulses from a point in the distal extremity (i.e. fingers) and conducts these impulses back to the spinal cord and brain to allow feeling.

Spasm

Continuous contraction of a muscle. This may result in pain and discomfort due to compression or pressure on nerves that travel through or beneath the muscle belly.

Splints

These are devices applied to an extremity which decrease motion. They are often helpful in calming down inflammation and treating nerve problems. They can be problematic if utilized inappropriately or if they cause a person to use an extremity in an abnormal manner attempting performance of activities in an abnormal way.

Surgeon

A physician who has further training in the techniques of surgical intervention. Surgeons also treat by conservative methods and when these fail, utilize surgery as one of many options to treat disease.

Symptoms

Those complaints a patient relates relative to the disease process. These may present as pain, swelling or numbness to name a few.

Synovitis

Inflammation of the lining structure of the moving units in the body.

Tendons

Tough semi-elastic cordlike structures which connect muscle to bone. They allow muscles to move bones and allow for finger motion as well as motion of the joints in the body.

Tenosynovitis

Inflammation of the surrounding tissues of tendons. When present in the carpal tunnel, this puts increased pressure on the median nerve resulting in early carpal tunnel nerve symptoms.

TENS (Transcutaneous Electrical Nerve Stimulation)

A form of therapeutic treatment which can be used in a therapy unit and at home. It essentially stimulates nerves to the point of exhaustion and decreases the amount of pain in some nerve problems. This may be highly effective in controlling nerve pain.

Therapist

A person trained in nonoperative, non-invasive techniques for treating and, hopefully, healing disease.

Thoracic Outlet Syndrome

Involves a myriad of symptoms. Patients classically have numbness, tingling, pain, and at times, motor dysfunction in the extremity. The involvement of the nerves is between the neck and shoulder at the area of the brachial plexus. These patients often have very confusing neurologic presentations with varied nerve distributions, exacerbated by various overhead positions of the arm. Symptoms may mimic those of many other nerve problems or syndromes in the upper extremity.

Tinel's Sign

A test done to elicit nerve pathology or inflammation. This is done by lightly tapping or lightly pressing on a nerve. If a reproduction of symptomatology is obtained, this indicates a positive test indicating inflammation and/or scarring about the nerve.

Traction Injury

A yanking or stretching injury which causes inflammation and sometimes tearing of the surrounding soft tissues about nerves. This results at times in pathologic scarring about these nerves. This often results in the production of numbness, tingling, and/or pain. This is a common mechanism for injury to the nerves of the brachial plexus, such as in whiplash, injuries to the neck, or yanking injuries on the arm.

Transverse Carpal Ligament

The structure which lies on the palm side of the carpal tunnel. This is a thick ligament or band which maintains the median nerve and the flexor tendons (which bend the fingers) inside the carpal canal. This ligament is opened during median nerve surgeries at the carpal tunnel.

Ulnar Nerve

The nerve which begins at the C-8 and T-1 nerve roots and travels down through the arm on the inside of the elbow (funny bone) and then travels down to the hand supplying the small and little finger side of the ring finger. It is also responsible for fine (intrinsic) function in the hand.

Ultrasound

A therapy modality utilizing sound waves to penetrate beneath the skin and heat the soft tissues. This is often helpful as a deep heat modality in decreasing inflammation, pain and discomfort.

Vein

Blood vessels which bring circulation back away from the extremities to the heart.

Whiplash

A term commonly used to indicate a forceful, traumatic injury to the neck and head. Most commonly associated with car accidents, although other injuries may result in the same. Whiplash injuries place tremendous stress on the ligament, disc, and muscle structures about the neck and also the nerves as they leave the neck in the way of nerve roots and the brachial plexus proper.

SUGGESTED REFERENCES & BIBLIOGRAPHY

Benson, Herbert M.D. *The Relaxation Response*. New York, NY: Avon Books, 1970.

————. *Beyond the Relaxation Response*. New York, NY: Berkeley Books.

Butler, Sharon J. *Conquering Carpal Tunnel Syndrome*. Oakland, CA: New Harbinger Publications.

Covey, Stephen. *The Seven Habits of Highly Effective People*. New York, NY: Simon and Schuster, A Fireside Book.

Crouch, Tammy. *Carpal Tunnel Syndrome and Repetitive Stress Injuries*. Berkeley, CA: Frog Ltd., distributed by North Atlantic Books.

"The Painful Hand." *Hand Clinics*, Edited by Roger Daley, M.D. and John Gould, M.D. Philadelphia, PA: W.B. Sanders and Co., November, 1996.

Hill, Napoleon. *Think and Grow Rich*. New York, NY: St. Martin's Press.

Hunter, James M.D., Evelyn Mackin, P.T., and Ann Callahan, M.S. *Rehabilitation of the Hand, Surgery and Therapy*, 4th ed. St. Louis, MO: Mosby - Yearbook, Inc.

Operative Hand Surgery. Edited by David P. Green, M.D. New York, NY: Churchill Livingstone.

Robbins, Anthony. *Power Talk.* A series of tapes: (1) Interview with Dr. Steven Covey; (2) Interview with Dr. Bernie Siegel. Los Angeles, CA: Audio Renaissance Tapes.

———. *Unlimited Power.* Ballantine Books, Fawcett Columbine Books.

Siegel, Bernie S. M.D. *Peace, Love and Healing.* New York, NY: Harper Perennial.

———. *Love Medicine and Miracles.* New York, NY: Harper and Row Publishers, Inc.

Sunderland, Sir Sydney. *Nerve Injuries and Their Repair.* New York, NY: Churchill Livingstone.

INDEX

A

Acupuncture 87
Adson, Dr. A.W. 140
Adson's Test 74-75
Aerobic exercises 175-176
Alternative medicines 154
Alternatives, future 171-179
Amyloidosis 43
Anesthesia, suggestion under 25
Anti-inflammatory medication 92
Antioxidants 173
Arthroscope 120
Autonomic instability 156
Axon 51

B

B-complex vitamins 173
Benson, Dr. Herbert 169
Beyond the Relaxation Response 169
Biofeedback 26, 88, 154, 159, 166
Biofeedback, hypnosis, and magic
  159-169
Bone spurs 76
Brachial plexus 13, 59, 130-133.
  See also Thoracic outlet
  syndrome

Brawny edema 156

C

Carpal tunnel, cross section diagram
  33
Carpal tunnel surgery, procedure for
  116-124
Carpal tunnel syndrome
  causes of 41-47
  conservative treatment 83-96
  description 33
  early stage symptoms 37
  early treatments 28
  incorrect diagnosis 32
  what is it? 31
Causalgia 151
Change, events occurring prior to 3
Checkers 46. *See also* repetitive
  activities
Chiropractic manipulation 89
Chronic disability 163
Cold modalities 87
Compression test 73
Computer use 2. *See also* Keyboard
  activities
Conservative treatment 83-96, 104
Cortisone 94